ROBYN TOOMATH works as a physician at Auckland City Hospital in New Zealand, where she is the clinical director of General Medicine. Early in her career as an endocrinologist she observed that her type 2 diabetes patients were both getting younger and increasing rapidly in numbers. Realizing that rising obesity was to blame, in 2001 she co-founded the advocacy group FOE (Fight the Obesity Epidemic) to raise awareness of this issue. As spokesperson for the organization Toomath has been constant in her call for a governmental response and public health measures to improve the obesogenic environment. She believes that making weight an issue of personal responsibility is not only ineffective but harmful to overweight individuals and has allowed industry to get off the hook. *The Obesity Epidemic* is the culmination of her work in this area, an effort to describe the real drivers of obesity in an in-depth and nuanced way. Toomath has also been the president of the New Zealand Society for the Study of Diabetes. She lives on Waiheke Island with her hens, Chrissie and Maisie.

The Obesity Epidemic

Why Diets and Exercise Don't Work—and What Does

Robyn Toomath

JOHNS HOPKINS UNIVERSITY PRESS | BALTIMORE

The moral rights of the author have been asserted.

First published in 2016 by Auckland University Press as *Fat Science:
Why Diets and Exercise Don't Work—and What Does*

Johns Hopkins University Press
2715 North Charles Street
Baltimore, Maryland 21218-4363
www.press.jhu.edu

Library of Congress Control Number: 2016949856
A catalog record for this book is available from the British Library.

ISBN 13: 978-1-4214-2249-7
ISBN 10: 1-4214-2249-2

*Special discounts are available for bulk purchases of this book. For more information,
please contact Special Sales at 410-516-6936 or specialsales@press.jhu.edu.*

Johns Hopkins University Press uses environmentally friendly book materials,
including recycled text paper that is composed of at least 30 percent
post-consumer waste, whenever possible.

To Robin White

Contents

Introduction

For more than 15 years I ran a private practice in Wellington whose patients included some of the city's most highly motivated and well-resourced individuals—lawyers, diplomats, doctors, and bankers. I am an endocrinologist and many of the patients referred to me were suffering from type 2 diabetes. Excess weight was the problem.

My patients were people used to having a high degree of control over their lives and were prepared to pay whatever money and put in whatever effort was required to manage their medical problems. 'Tell me what weight you want me to be, Doc, and I'll get there' was a typical response. Others had spent half their lives on diets and were less optimistic about losing weight, but most were willing to give it another go. They promised to join a gym, get a dog to take walking or play more tennis, and to eat well.

At the end of the initial consultation the patient and I were both filled with purpose and optimism.

Three months later, most patients reported a drop in weight, an improvement in blood sugar levels, and an overall feeling of increased health and energy. We celebrated the changes and looked forward to more.

Sometimes things kept going well. But more often my patients' weight started to creep up again. By 12 months most had started to regain weight and some just stopped showing up at the clinic, ashamed of their failure. By two years almost all had returned to their original weight.

What happened next? A few were persuaded to have gastric bypass surgery. Others resigned themselves to the inevitable, and our focus shifted to managing the diabetes, high blood pressure, and raised cholesterol with medication.

Over the same period, I ran a diabetes clinic for teenagers. As time went on the numbers of teenagers with type 2 diabetes increased. As with adults, the key for them was to lose excess weight. They were growing children with high energy requirements so losing weight should have been easy. If you keep their energy intake to a certain level, children should become slim.

Well, maybe. One of my teenage patients was a 14-year-old girl who weighed more than 300 pounds at the time her diabetes was diagnosed. She was intelligent, engaged, and desperately keen to be slim. She wanted to avoid insulin injections, but this paled into insignificance alongside worries about self-esteem and peer pressure. We set up dietician appointments, talked about her physical activity (which was actually very high—she played a lot of sports), and moaned about her big-eating older brothers.

I scheduled follow-up appointments and she attended most of them. Astonishingly, at every appointment she was heavier than at the last—her weight increasing in parallel with her growth in height. She completed school, and by the time she finished a law degree she was on insulin therapy, anti-hypertensive drugs, and cholesterol-lowering drugs. By then we were planning gastric bypass surgery.

Television programs such as *The Biggest Loser* and thousands of magazine articles tell us that we can lose weight by following this new diet or adopting that exciting exercise regime. When patients came to see me in the clinic I gave them much the same advice.

But my years of experience, treating the same individuals, gradually changed my attitude. I realized that asking people to lose a significant amount of weight and keep it off was about as useful as asking them to change their eye color. No other therapeutic strategy employed in medicine has such poor results so why was I continuing to prescribe it? Not only was the treatment I was recommending ineffective but it was my patient who was invariably left with the sense of failure. Inducing a sense of guilt or hopelessness doesn't fit with my understanding of the Hippocratic Oath. So, years ago, I made the decision to stop asking patients to lose weight.

This book is for the people (and their spouses, their children, their parents, and their doctors too) who try to lose weight but fail. It's for the overweight people who think it's all their fault. If we really want to tackle the problems that come with obesity we first need to understand why most of us can't change our body size. In Part 1 I look at the conventional (and a few unconventional) approaches to weight loss and consider how successful these really are. Scientific study tells us that our own efforts following diets, heading to the gym, or taking some new pills are defeated again and again by our genes. Placing responsibility for weight control on individuals suits the food industry, which claims that their responsibility with regard to the obesity epidemic extends no further than providing choice. And it suits governments, who like to avoid putting in place regulations that restrict the free market. But, as we will learn, the drivers of obesity lie outside the control of individuals.

So why are we getting fatter? Why are more young people developing what we used to call maturity onset (type 2) diabetes? In Part 2 I turn my attention to the true drivers of the obesity epidemic—how the world we live in is making us fat. I examine how the changes in our environment—our physical world, the economics of food, the role of marketing, rising inequality—determine what we eat and how much we exercise.

I think we now know what's causing the problem. But do we also know how to fix it? In Part 3, I first look at the role of government—because government does have a key role. Internationally, changes in governmental policy have led to just the sorts of behavioral shifts that will end the obesity epidemic. On the other hand there are many, many examples of governments doing very little. Second, I look at the role of you and me. While it might be easier to get people to rally around a single issue like bicycle helmets or gun control, increasingly I think that civil unrest may be the only way to fix obesity.

Yes, it's true that ultimately we decide what to eat, but what is it that makes some of us turn so easily to a packet of chips and others an apple? I would like to put an end to the myth of personal responsibility for body size. And I would like overweight people to feel entitled to an environment which makes it easier, not harder, to remain healthy and slim. Eating healthy food and getting enough exercise should be the default, not something we have to battle for.

PART 1

We all want to be thin. Why aren't we?

1

Does dieting work?

'How did I let this happen again?'

Oprah Winfrey is the doyenne of self-empowerment. Legions
of fans celebrate her achievements yet in 2008 she wrote in her
magazine, *O*:

> In 1992 I reached my heaviest, 237 pounds. I was 38. Then, four years
> ago, I made it a goal to lose weight, and I appeared on the January
> 2005 cover at a toned 160 pounds. I thought I was finished with the
> weight battle. I was done. I'd conquered it. I was so sure, I was even
> cocky. I had the nerve to say to friends who were struggling, 'All you
> have to do is work out harder and eat less! Get your 10,000 steps in!
> None of that starchy stuff!'
>
>   *Bam!* Karma is a bear of a thing.
>
>   So here I stand, 40 pounds heavier than I was in 2006. (Yes, you're
> adding correctly; that means the dreaded 2-0-0.) I'm mad at myself.

I'm embarrassed. I can't believe that after all these years, all the things I know how to do, I'm still talking about my weight. I look at my thinner self and think, 'How did I let this happen again?'

Oprah's explanation for her weight regain in 2008 was that she had an underactive thyroid gland. But correcting this easily treated problem didn't result in weight loss and soon she was back on the Better Body Bootcamp. If someone like Oprah battles obesity, despite having personal chefs preparing her meals and a dedicated weight loss trainer, what hope is there for mere mortals?

Everybody is dieting

In the United States market researchers estimated that the weight loss market was worth $121 billion in 2009 and predicted to reach $206.4 billion by 2019.[1] In Finland, 36% of healthy adults surveyed said they were trying to lose weight.[2] In Britain marketing agency Mintel surveyed Britons at the beginning of 2014 and found that 65% of women and 44% of men had tried to lose weight over the previous year.[3]

The law of thermodynamics applies to the human body—in order to lose weight you need to put less energy in than energy out. But simply eating less is hard. So diets typically tell their adherents to follow some highly prescribed regime of restricted eating. The Israeli Army diet consists of two days of eating just apples, two days of cheese, two days of chicken and two days of salad, after which you presumably start again. The Beverley Hills diet requires you to eat nothing but fruit for the first 10 days.

There's the seven-day cabbage soup diet, a complicated regime of unlimited soup and water in combination with low calorie foods that vary from day to day. It's a near-starvation diet that produces a lot of gas. There's the Atkins diet, which aims at zero carbohydrates while allowing people to continue to eat many of their favourite high-fat foods.[4] And currently popular is the paleo or caveman diet, whose followers avoid processed foods, sugars, and grains like wheat. Skeptics point out that humans have been cooking wild corn, tubers and legumes for at least 400,000 years, and that a proper paleo diet would involve eating rats, mice, frogs, and a mass of insects, but it seems there are very few purists out there.

Such diets can have some short-term success. That success is probably due to the severe restriction of the range of foods available to eat, and perhaps the monotony of the diet helping to suppress appetite.

But humans are obligate omnivores—we are designed to forage widely, and to eat a large variety of plants and animals to fulfil our body's requirements for trace elements. Restrictive diets don't allow that. A study of women attempting weight loss using different diets found that at eight weeks many had inadequate intakes of micronutrients. On the Atkins diet subjects were short of thiamine, folate, vitamin C, iron and magnesium; on the LEARN (Lifestyle, Exercise, Attitudes, Relationships, Nutrition) diet it was vitamin E, thiamine and magnesium; and on the low-fat Ornish diet vitamins E, B12 and zinc were lacking.[5]

Such nutrient deficiency poses real risk. Some hospital-based physicians and dieticians prescribe what is known as the very low calorie diet. The diet limits energy intake to 400–800 calories a day, rather than the 2000 calories usually required by a relatively sedentary female. When the very low calorie diet was first used in the 1970s, there were reports of sudden death related to protein, vitamin, and mineral deficiencies. In the United States 60 people died from cardiac problems after an average of four months dieting and 30% weight loss.[6] Many obese individuals have heart disease, some of which persists after losing weight. If you add nutritional deficiencies, particularly of copper, potassium, and magnesium, electrical instability in the heart can trigger a fatal heart rhythm. These days physicians supplement such diets with micronutrients to make them safe. Depending on the diet, calories are fixed at between 400 and 800 a day, and the diets are used to achieve particular outcomes, such as shrinking the liver by reducing its fat content in preparation for gastric bypass and other abdominal surgery. For those who can adhere to them, these diets produce quite fast weight loss, but over six months or so they are no more effective than a low calorie diet of 1000 calories a day because the former is so difficult to stick to.

The dangers of nutrient deficiency in many extreme diets mean that none of these regimes is suitable for long-term use. Fortunately, or unfortunately, long-term use is unlikely because people struggle to stick to any of these extreme diets. The more extreme, the less the adherence. A study that compared the Atkins diet to the more balanced Weight Watchers, Zone, and Ornish diets found that both adherence to the diet and weight loss was lowest with the Atkins.[7]

Diets to improve overall health as well as assist weight loss have been popular since the mid-twentieth century. In 1956 the New York City Department of Health, Bureau of Nutrition set up the Anti-Coronary Club and developed the Prudent diet designed to reduce heart disease through lowering cholesterol. This was one of the first low-fat diets. The Mediterranean diet, popularized in the 1970s, was designed to mimic the eating patterns from a region of the world where the population has a low rate of heart disease despite relatively high smoking rates. In 1983 the F-Plan diet book was a bestseller in the United States. This described a high-fiber regimen promoted as a healthy diet that would make you feel full for longer. Unfortunately it also produced a lot of flatulence and constipation. In 1995 the biochemist Barry Sears invented the Zone diet with strict proportions of carbohydrates, protein and fat. This was in response to his father dying early of a heart attack, but the diet is a low calorie one designed to reduce weight as well as cardiac disease.

Over time the art of restricting calories while leaving the dieter feeling full has become more sophisticated with the help of research into eating behavior. Professor Barbara Rolls developed the Volumetric diet as a result of studies with adults and children showing satiety is a response more to volume than to calories. The most effective way to maintain volume while decreasing calories is to add water. So the recommendation is to eat soups and stews with lots of vegetables.[8] Interestingly, another study demonstrated that drinking water *with* food didn't really make a difference and the water really had to be *within* food in order to contribute to satiety. This sort of diet is inherently healthy, and in many ways mimics a traditional diet which is high in volume and fibre, and of low calorie density.

But all that dieting isn't working

A quick search on Google reveals thousands of papers reporting successful weight loss in response to one diet or another. If we look more carefully, though, many are studies lasting a few weeks or a few months. What are the results like over a longer period?

In 2000, Danish researchers reviewed studies published between 1931 and 1999 to assess the long-term impact of diets on obesity. They looked for papers that followed up patients for three years or more and included at least 50% of the original subjects at the end of the study. Of the 898 papers, only 17 met the criteria. What did those long-term studies show? Of the 3,030 patients studied in the papers, 15% achieved significant weight loss, losing 19 pounds or more. For the other 85%, the weight loss at three years or longer was less than 19 pounds. Many of these people would have been heavier at the end of the period than they were at the start.[9] Nevertheless, on average people in such studies do lose weight. A second similar study suggested that for those who participate in a structured weight loss program the average person is still about 6 pounds lighter after five years than they were at the start. But the weight loss flattens out year by year. Of the original weight lost, 67% is still off at one year, 44% at two years, 32% at three years, 28% at four years and 21% at five years.[10]

One of the most comprehensive recent studies of the effect of dieting showed similar results. The Look AHEAD (Action for Health in Diabetes) study started out with 5,145 overweight or obese people with type 2 diabetes and put them into either an intensive lifestyle intervention (ILI) or 'usual care', which meant receiving three group educational sessions a year on diet and exercise. The first group did better. At the end of four years 372 had maintained weight loss of greater than 10%. By my reckoning this means that 4,771 failed to achieve meaningful weight loss (for example from 220 to 200 pounds). These were highly moti-vated individuals (after all, they had volunteered for a weight loss study), but after four years 45% of the usual care and 26% of the ILI groups had gained weight.[11]

Even these results oversell the effectiveness of the program. In a regular therapeutic trial, the results are collected from everyone who enters the trial—whether they got better or didn't, whether they took the drug in question or didn't. If the results of weight loss studies were analyzed in the same way, all patients who enrolled at the beginning would be weighed at the five year mark. But in practice only those who stick with the program are studied, which inevitably biases the results towards success. For example, a commercial weight loss program was reported to be very successful at 24 months when used by a group of individuals who were offered all sorts of incentives including free participation. The same program was subsequently used in a much larger study and of the 60,164 women who enrolled only 7% remained in the program at one year. High attrition distorts the outcome for just about every weight loss initiative that you read about.[12]

If efforts focused on individuals don't really seem to work, what happens when the focus is on changing a whole community? From 1980 to 1993, in three cities, the Minnesota Heart Health Program established courses, seminars and workshops for the general population, and school-based programs for school children and their parents, all designed to improve cardiovascular health. Those three cities were subsequently compared to three similar cities who served as the reference population.[13] At every measurement point between 1980 and 2000, the body mass index (BMI) of the populations of the three participating cities steadily rose from around 24.5 for women at the outset to 27.5 at the end, with a comparable rise for men. This was identical to the communities who had received no education. I can remember the epidemiologist Robert Jeffery presenting the findings at a conference—he described his profound disappointment at the results. He suggested several reasons for their complete lack of success, ranging from overwhelming commercial influences promoting the consumption of a high calorie diet to failure in the design of the intervention. Perhaps the most plausible reason, he suggested, was a ceiling effect—that everyone who needed to lose weight was already trying to do so and that the population was already saturated with information before they started.[14]

Community-based weight loss projects for children have seen some success. In Colac, a small city southwest of Melbourne, the Be Active, Eat Well initiative was a whole-of-community pilot study aimed at 4–12-year-olds. At the end of the study the children weighed about 2 pounds less and had a smaller waist measurement. But this occurred not only in the targeted communities but also in the neighboring control groups.[15] In New Zealand, the Project Energize program has been designed to improve nutrition and increase physical activity in primary and intermediate school children. At last report 44,000 children in hundreds of schools across the Waikato were enrolled. When evaluated in 2014 they found that obesity rates were 3% less than the national average and the children were also more physically fit.[16]

But overall the evidence seems clear. For the great majority, dieting as a means of achieving lasting weight reduction just doesn't work. Of course, in among the failures are some outstanding successes. It's a bit like buying Lotto tickets; for those who win it is a stunningly successful strategy. But most of us wouldn't advocate Lotto as a way of securing a financially stable future. The odds of success from dieting are in fact a bit better than winning Lotto, and for certain groups there is evidence that some strategies may be effective.

Everybody may be dieting but we are not getting any thinner. In May 2014, figures from the Global Burden of Disease Study showed a 47.1% rise in childhood obesity and a 27.5% increase in adult obesity between 1980 and 2013.[17] You would think from Oprah's outburst of frustration that her failure to stay slim after losing weight was unusual. But the real surprise is that anyone who ever loses weight keeps it off. Why?

Fighting our own physiology

For centuries, humans struggled to avoid starvation. Now we struggle to avoid obesity. In a world where science has provided the answers to many questions, the obesity problem has proved remarkably intractable. Part of the difficulty is that we underestimate what we're up against, and embark on efforts to lose weight with unreasonable optimism. No matter what diet we try, our bodies are singularly resistant to giving up stores of fat.

When it comes to losing weight, the biggest battle is with our own physiology. The human body is maintained by a myriad of homeostatic mechanisms that keep things in balance. When we move from lying to standing, the nervous system immediately adjusts, increasing our heart rate and blood pressure to maintain blood flow to the brain. Hormones released from the heart, in response to changes in pressure in the ventricles, signal the kidneys, altering the reabsorption of salt and water so that blood volume and salt levels are kept constant. So too with body weight—except in this case the balancing isn't very precise, and is heavily skewed in favor of weight gain. Evolution, in the face of scarce food, has equipped us with powerful mechanisms to avoid starvation. Our body's physiology is less agile at responding to the threat of obesity.

The signalling mechanism for food intake and energy storage is complicated and relies on the brain integrating a number of hormonal messages. Some of these come from fat itself. Fat cells are not just inert storage containers. They are highly active metabolically and, among other things, they make leptin. This hormone has a direct effect on the hypothalamus, the area of the brain that controls some of our most basic behaviours, including the drive to eat and drink. Leptin is the hormone that should keep us from getting fat. As fat increases, leptin levels rise and they tell the brain to stop eating. But the signal is relatively weak. Leptin is also important for reproduction, telling the brain that a woman is sufficiently well nourished for a successful pregnancy. Once the fat mass, and therefore leptin, reaches a certain level, the hypothalamus releases fertility hormones and the ovaries once again produce eggs. Accordingly, in times of extreme starvation most women are infertile.

Insulin, another key hormone controlling what we eat, is more sensitive to food *intake* than to the level of energy already stored. That is why a day of calorie restriction will result in a powerful drive to eat, irrespective of our fat stores. You may weigh 550 pounds, but if one day you eat only 500 calories your insulin hormones will signal that you are at risk of starving to death.

Meanwhile, ghrelin, sometimes called the 'hunger hormone,' works through the hypothalamus to *stimulate* eating. Blood levels of this hormone rise when we are hungry, signalling when we should eat, and fall after we have eaten. People with the genetic

disorder Prader-Willi syndrome are obese as a result of their voracious appetite, and it appears that part of the problem is that they
have higher than normal ghrelin levels. However, the story with
ghrelin is complicated and most obese people have lower ghrelin
levels than do thin people; so ghrelin can't be a direct cause of
obesity. But the fact that ghrelin levels rise when calories are
restricted means that this hormone plays a role in making weight
loss more difficult.[18]

A further, crucial part of the story is the relationship between
hormone levels and the number of fat cells. This number is determined by genes and nutrition in intra-uterine and early childhood
and is set from that time onwards. Although about 8% of cells turn
over each year, the number doesn't change and the individual
cells expand and shrink when we gain or lose weight. Two people
may be equally fat with one having lots of small cells and the other
few large cells. The smaller a fat cell, the less leptin it produces
(so less signals to the hypothalamus telling us that we are full) and
the more sensitive it is to insulin (which drives fat storage). So a
person who starts out with a lot of fat cells is going to suffer more
from the hormone changes that encourage weight regain than
someone with fewer.

But it seems as if all fat cells are not the same when it comes
to hormonal signalling. Liposuction removes large numbers of
subcutaneous fat cells but there is no improvement in insulin
resistance or any other measures of metabolic problems associated with obesity. This is probably because fat in the abdominal
cavity releases free fatty acids into the blood that feeds into the
liver. The liver responds to this with additional hormones to
restrict weight gain but with the side effect of insulin resistance
so the adverse metabolic effects of fat are amplified.

As well as hormonally driven appetite and satiety (energy in), the physiology of energy expenditure (energy out) matters for weight gain and loss. If you successfully lose weight your energy requirements fall. This is the most important factor driving weight regain. About 80% of our energy requirements is to fuel basic body processes such as breathing, heart pumping, digestion, cell metabolism and tissue repair. Tissues vary widely in their energy demands with the brain being the heaviest user, taking up to 20% of the total to fire electrical impulses and maintain cellular function. This is known as our resting energy expenditure. When we lose weight there is a significant fall in the required resting energy expenditure. Most of this is due to the loss of muscle tissue, which has high energy demands, rather than to the loss of fat. In addition, because more energy is required to move around 220 pounds (for example) than 200 pounds, *exercise-related* energy expenditure also decreases. The third problem is that when you are starved you probably do less in order to conserve energy. In calorie-deprived lab rats you certainly see a compensatory decrease in voluntary physical activity.[19] One of the frustrations of physiology is that losing weight means you need to keep putting in less energy.

Regardless of the underlying biological mechanisms, what we experience as a calorie- restricted individual is *hunger*. A 12-week study during which the subjects had a 25% restriction in calorie intake resulted in a loss of weight, a loss of fat mass, a reduction in metabolic rate and a sharp increase in hunger.[20] Hunger didn't decline over the 12 weeks of the study. Other experiments have shown that following a period of limiting calories people usually overeat. In one experiment, participants were restricted to 50% of energy requirements for a period of 24 weeks, followed by eight weeks of 75% of energy requirements, then 12 weeks of unrestricted eating. The overeating that occurred in the final period saw some of the study subjects consuming 160% of their daily energy requirements, and this went on well after they had regained the fat they had lost. The reason for this is clear—it's not a question of habits (or greed). The hormones that drive weight regain don't reset when you have lost weight. A study performed 62 weeks after participants took up a weight loss program showed persistent hunger in its subjects compared to the baseline.[21]

The Darwinian theory of survival of the fittest (fattest) has selected for genes which encourage energy storage. Those who avidly seek out food are more likely to survive in times of famine and if they live to reproductive age will also have a higher chance of being sufficiently well nourished to be fertile. This results in an enrichment of 'starvation avoidance' genes being passed on to the next generation. Only in recent times are we seeing a survival *disadvantage* associated with being overweight, in the form of early deaths from heart disease and cancer. This won't affect the gene pool, though, until being overweight reduces fertility. Fortunately the prevalence of obesity in our reproductive years is still relatively low with weight peaking on average in our sixties; genetic adaptation is a long way off.

So does anything work?

The best example of a successful weight loss intervention that I know of is the Finnish Diabetes Prevention Study (DPS). This 10-year study recruited volunteers through local advertisements or from other epidemiological studies. The volunteers had to be between 40 and 64 years of age, with a BMI greater than 25 (overweight), and to have slightly high blood sugar levels. The aim with these pre-diabetes people was to prevent them from progressing to type 2 diabetes.

The researchers asked the participants to achieve five things—to reduce their weight by at least 5%; to undertake moderately intense activity for at least 30 minutes each day; to reduce dietary fat to less than 30% of total energy; to reduce saturated fat to less than 10% of total energy; and to include at least 15 grams of fiber for every 1,000 kilocalories per day. A control group and the intervention group received the same advice but in addition the intervention group had seven sessions with a nutritionist over the first year of the study, and quarterly individual visits thereafter. They also had teaching sessions, such as visits to the supermarket and cooking lessons, and they received follow-up phone calls and written material. Food diaries kept over a three-day period were analyzed four times a year, and specific advice was given based on the results. If the supervisors of the study thought a participant's weight loss was too slow after six months, they could have several weeks of a very low calorie diet meal replacement. They were offered free supervised exercise classes and voluntary group hiking and walking activities. Several centers ran exercise competitions to increase motivation in the study participants.

The results were moderately encouraging. At the end of the 2.8-year randomized trial the intervention group had an initial 58% reduction in the rate of progression to type 2 diabetes when compared to the control group, and this was associated with modest weight loss (about 8 pounds at the end of year two compared to about 2 pounds in the control group).[22] Subsequent reports have shown that ten years out from original randomization the intensive lifestyle group had partially regained the weight they had lost but still had 34% less diabetes than the control group. The rate of new diabetes year on year wasn't different, though, with another 5.9 cases per 100 person years in the treatment group and 5.6 cases in the placebo group.[23] In China, a similar study ran for six years. Twenty years later 80% of those in the study group, and 93% of the control group, had gone on to develop diabetes.[24]

These two studies required huge resources from government and huge commitment from participants. While they had some impact on weight and diabetes, could they be replicated beyond a small study population? Isn't that expecting everyone to live like Oprah—with personal chefs and personalized exercise and diet regimes? And we know how well Oprah did: '*Bam!* Karma is a bear of a thing.' If diets don't work, then what does?

2

Is exercise the answer?

No one doubts that exercise is good for us. Humans evolved from hunter-gatherers who spent most of the day in physical activity. Keeping active is important for psychological wellbeing, regular bowel activity, good sleep, muscle strength, co-ordination, and balance. It also protects us from the metabolic syndrome, that terrible combination of susceptibility to easy weight gain, particularly around the middle, high blood pressure, heart disease and fatty liver as well as obesity. But can we use exercise as a tool to lose weight? Or is it like diet—where some of us are more naturally inclined to be physically active, and the environment in which we live will either aid or impede behavior?

I know I'm lucky—eternally (infuriatingly) busy by nature and I can do an hour of fast walking a day just getting to work and back. I don't do any other form of exercise. It wasn't always like this though. When my children were small I spent all my spare time with them. We lived driving distance from the hospital where I worked and for years I didn't do any regular exercise. If exercise had been prescribed for me by my doctor I would have failed to comply.

The commitment to losing weight through exercise is enormous. The investment is made by individuals who want to lose weight as well as the huge exercise industry, including gyms, personal trainers, sports equipment and specialized clothing and footwear companies. But it's also supported by the fast food and soft drinks industries. Sponsorship of sports is a great way to promote an unhealthy product and emphasizing the benefits of physical activity also deflects attention from diet as a cause of obesity. Governments like it, too, because it's easier to promote sports than to regulate the food environment.

But how good is exercise as a means of losing weight? Is one form better than another for weight loss, for other aspects of health? Do we know what a healthy amount of exercise is? Are we doing it? If not, why not?

Is exercise an effective way to lose weight?

The theory is simple. Weight balance is a matter of energy in and energy out. The Mayo Clinic produced a chart listing 32 different forms of exercise and the number of calories burned if you did these for an hour, adjusted according to body weight (because the heavier you are, the more calories you burn).[1] They also state that you need an energy deficit of 3,500 calories to lose 1 pound (0.45 kilograms). According to their chart, all you need do is decide how much weight you want to lose, choose something you like doing, do it for the requisite period of time, and bingo! You are the right weight. For example, someone weighing 240 pounds might need to lose about 66 pounds. This equates to walking at 2 miles (3.2 kilometers) an hour for 765 hours (or 63 days if you walk for just 12 hours a day). Assuming, of course, that the exercise doesn't make you hungry and want to eat more.

Weight of person and calories burned per hour

	160 lb	200 lb	240 lb
Aerobics	533	664	796
Ballroom dancing	219	273	327
Bicycling (leisurely)	292	364	436
Canoeing	256	319	382
Cross training	365	455	545
Football (touch)	584	728	872
Golf (carry clubs)	314	391	469
Running, 5 mph	606	755	905
Running, 8 mph	861	1074	1286
Skiing downhill	314	391	469
Swimming, laps	423	528	632
Tai chi	219	273	327
Tennis, singles	584	728	872
Walking, 2 mph	204	255	305
Walking, 3.5 mph	314	391	469
Yoga, hatha	183	228	273

Adapted by the Mayo Clinic from: B. E. Ainsworth, et al. '2011 compendium of physical activities: A second update of codes and MET values.' *Medicine and Science in Sports and Exercise* vol. 43, 2011, p. 1575.

It makes more sense to combine calorie restriction and moderate exercise to attain an energy deficit. Lots of short-term studies confirm that this works (actually pretty well everything works in the short term) as do a few which tease out the effects of exercise from dieting.

One study divided participants into diet-induced weight loss, exercise-induced weight loss, exercise without weight loss, and control groups. After three months both weight loss groups had dropped an average of 16.5 pounds. Other researchers looked at overweight and obese volunteers in a longer study of aerobic exercise, without dietary restriction. People were randomized to a 400 kilocalorie per session, a 600 kilocalorie per session or a no-exercise control group for five supervised sessions a week for 10 months. At the end of the 10 months the weight changes for the three groups were 4.3% weight loss, 5.7% weight loss and 0.5% weight gain, respectively.

On face value these results look good and suggest doctors should recommend such an exercise program for weight loss. But let's look at the study in more detail. The investigators assessed 2,338 volunteers but only 141 people were deemed suitable for inclusion. They excluded people with hypertension, diabetes, or another chronic disease and those with modestly elevated blood pressure, lipids, or blood sugar. They excluded smokers and anyone on medication likely to affect their sporting performance or metabolism. And they excluded those who were already doing a reasonable amount of exercise. Once in the study, the participants had to attend 90% or more of the exercise sessions or they were out. That took out another 49 participants, leaving just 92. Unlike the real world, where you pay to attend exercise classes, subjects *received* payment to attend.[2] Finally, we need to remember that if the exercise program is anything like the dieting regimes, success at 10 months is no guarantee of long-term weight loss.

So while this study clarified, in a highly refined group of individuals, the short-term effect of exercise without dieting on weight, it seems highly unlikely that these results are transferable to the general population. Most people needing to lose weight for health reasons would never have been accepted for this study.

Is one form of exercise better than another for weight loss? Many papers promote the benefit of high intensity or low, aerobic or resistance. I think the number of studies supporting one form of exercise over another cancel each other out and the bottom line is that it's the quantity of energy that matters: the more you burn, the more weight you lose and the more your overall health benefits (independent of weight loss). One study compared appetite and energy intake in healthy individuals who were asked to perform continuous exercise one week and an energy-equivalent short bout of high-intensity exercise another. They found both forms of exercise were equally effective means of producing an energy deficit.[3]

The bigger issue is that changing the amount of recreational or optional exercise we do is very difficult to sustain. Like anyone, I can think of people who have become hooked on marathon running or cycling and dramatically improved their health as a result, but these people are exceptions.

So are we exercising?

Repetitive or extreme exercise is damaging but most of us risk harm as a result of inactivity. The World Health Organization (WHO) states that more active people have lower rates of all-cause mortality, coronary heart disease, high blood pressure, stroke, type 2 diabetes, metabolic syndrome, colon and breast cancer, and depression. Experts considered the evidence and provided guidelines for minimum levels of physical activity.

For children aged 5–17 years the recommendation is at least 60 minutes of moderate to vigorous activity a day—including activities likely to build bone and muscle. The aim is to develop healthy musculoskeletal tissues (bones, muscles, and joints); a healthy cardiovascular system (heart and lungs); neuromuscular awareness (co-ordination and movement control); and lastly to facilitate maintenance of a healthy body weight.

For adults aged 18–65 the recommendations are for at least 150 minutes of moderate-intensity aerobic physical activity a week or at least 75 minutes of vigorous-intensity aerobic physical activity a week.

For adults aged 65 and over the recommendations are the same as for younger adults in terms of duration with an added recommendation that aerobic exercise is performed in 10 minute bursts. The relationship of exercise to improved health is probably stronger in this group and, if possible, older adults are advised to aim for 300 minutes of exercise a week and to include muscle-strengthening exercises.[4]

These sound eminently sensible. So are we doing it? WHO (again) estimates that physical inactivity causes 1.9 million deaths a year worldwide (this figure includes the contribution to breast and colon cancer as well as to cardiovascular disease). So the answer is NO. Carol Propper is Professor of Economics at Imperial College Business School, London, with a particular interest in the economics of health. She and researchers from Bristol University reported on a physical activity survey showing 80% of Britons fail to exercise enough. For some the inactivity is extreme. About 8% of those physically capable of walking hadn't even done so for five minutes continuously in the last month while almost half (46%) hadn't walked for leisure for 30 minutes in the last month. Individuals with higher education, more wealth and those living nearer sports facilities were more likely to be regular exercisers.[5]

An older study of US citizens indicated that as many as 47% of the population met recommendations for recreational exercise but again there was a strong relationship with this and levels of education. Physical disability, which is linked to age, ethnicity and, again, socio-economic status, is part of the problem. Overall 15% of the population said they were unable to perform physical activities such as walk a quarter of a mile or climb 10 steps without resting. Disability is more common in women compared to men, in black people compared to white, and in poor compared to wealthy.[6]

Can we change exercise levels?

Scottish researchers tried to increase physical activity and reduce BMI in a large group of preschool children using an enhanced physical activity program of 30 minutes' duration, three times a week. They used an accelerometer, which is like a pedometer but more sensitive to the erratic activity of toddlers and young children. The target was preschoolers because in Scotland 10% of children aged 4–5 and 20% of 11–12-year-olds are already obese. But assessment at the end of the 24 week intervention found no difference in activity levels or BMI between the study and the control group.[7]

The result was surprising and the researchers wondered if they should have tried harder with the exercise. But the explanation may be that physical activity is almost as immutable as weight. The endocrinologist Professor Wilkin measured physical activity in young children in Plymouth, again using accelerometers, and found that activity was more or less independent of factors like physical education at school and seemed to be controlled by a centrally acting 'set point'. He compared 9-year-olds from different types of school—a private school with extensive sporting facilities, a village school with a focus on physical activity, and an inner-city school with no particular emphasis or facilities. He also studied a group of children in Glasgow, about as different in diet, culture, and climate as you can get from Plymouth. He found that environment had almost no effect on physical activity levels which stayed constant for an individual from one day to another. Despite very different physical environments, activity levels were within 0.3% of each other for children from Glasgow and Plymouth. Despite a five-fold difference in school-based physical activity this had no effect overall because the behavior of the kids outside school compensated for it. Similarly, the impact of walking to school versus being driven was eliminated by other forms of physical activity. Activity for an individual child didn't change from weekday to weekend or from summer to winter. So while some children are definitely more active than others, and this is constant for that child, the only group difference was that girls were less active than boys.[8]

This is very important data which is largely ignored. It suggests that using incentives or motivating children to be more physically active (in this current environment) is harder than you think. Not impossible though. Project Energize has successfully increased exercise levels with demonstrable improvements in physical fitness and some loss of weight. This is a 'whole of school, and whole of health' program that includes improved nutrition as well as emphasizing physical activity.[9]

But changing patterns of exercise is very tough. Studies show that non-recreational exercise may be more important—the energy expended at work or getting to and from work. In 1953 a paper in *The Lancet* described the prevalence of coronary heart disease in London Transport workers. For the drivers, who spent most of their shift sitting down, the rate of cardiac events was roughly twice that of the conductors who pounded up and down between the bus's top and bottom decks.[10] A more recent UK study examined the mode of transport people used to get to work and correlated this with body weights for 20,000 individuals across England, Scotland, and Wales. Researchers discovered several interesting findings—the first is that relatively few people use active transport with 69% of the group travelling to work by car. Only 16% used public transport, 12% walked and 3% cycled.[11] Those using public transport were less likely to be overweight than car drivers, those who walked or cycled were less likely to have diabetes and those who walked were less likely to be hypertensive. These findings seem to be 'dose-dependent,' in that you had to walk a minimum distance (2 miles) in order to get the benefit of walking and a Finnish study found that cycling reduced the risk of diabetes once you cycled for 30 minutes or more.[12] With public transport, of course, the bus or train tends not to leave from outside your house and deliver you to the door of your workplace, and a US study found that on average people who used public transport walked for 19 minutes a day so the advantage comes from this part of the journey.[13]

Lately scientists have begun to wonder whether the link between physical inactivity and obesity-related diseases is more complicated than an imbalance in the energy equation. Are there dangers specifically associated with extreme inactivity—for example, spending the entire day sitting at a desk, as many of us do? It appears that this is the case. Sedentary behavior is now defined as sitting or lying while awake and using only slightly more energy than the basal metabolic requirements. As sedentary behavior goes up, so does obesity, cancer, type 2 diabetes, and death from cardiovascular disease. This is because physiological processes such as the absorption of fats and generation of healthy lipids, which are important for preventing insulin resistance, are switched off when muscles are completely quiescent. Only a light amount of activity is required to keep these processes ticking over and perhaps this is why exercise is so effective in improving or preventing type 2 diabetes even if we don't lose weight.

A group from the Baker Institute in Melbourne, which specializes in obesity, diabetes, and cardiovascular research, are behind a program called Stand Up Australia. Rather than encouraging more vigorous activity they suggest standing computer workstations in order to decrease sitting time.[14] A pilot study showed a decrease in lipid levels when subjects' computer desks were replaced with standing workstations, but the study also saw some compensation for standing with decreased activity outside work, just like the accelerometer studies with children. The intervention group decreased their sitting time at work by 143 minutes but only by 97 minutes over the entire day. The results were maintained at three months and this was enough to produce a statistically significant increase in the levels of healthy (protective) HDL cholesterol.[15]

Another hint that reducing inactivity has benefits independent of the quantum of exercise performed in a day comes from a small study in which 70 healthy weight individuals were required to either sit for nine hours, or to take part in 30 minutes of exercise prior to sitting for nine hours, or to have the equivalent activity divided up into short bursts every half an hour. They found that intermittent exercise was more effective than continuous exercise in lowering the diabetes markers of post-meal insulin, blood glucose, and triglyceride levels.[16] These participants were all healthy, normal weight individuals, and it will be interesting to see the study repeated in those with type 2 diabetes for whom the benefits may be greater.

The person best able to sum up all this information is Professor Adrian Bauman from the University of Sydney. He has written on every aspect of physical activity and health, and in 2013 he and others were asked to produce a review of whole-of-government obesity prevention interventions for the federal government in Australia. With respect to physical activity Bauman wrote that 'the evidence around regulatory or legislative strategies to promote physical activity and active transport are limited, with most of the published literature being conceptual rather than evaluations of interventions.' Despite the limitations the group came up with recommendations that were clustered around aspects of urban design, such as the provision of walking and cycling trails and parks, and the promotion of active transport and workplace interventions.[17]

As with nutrition, making the default environment conducive to physical activity is going to be more successful than imploring individuals to join gyms or increase recreational activity in other ways. Bauman's other work bears out the fact that recreational activity isn't where the money is. He looked at self-reported physical activity levels over a wide range of countries and New Zealand rated highest in the 'high physical activity' grouping, with 63% of the population stating that they were very physically active (playing sports, going to the gym) several days a week. Yet New Zealand is ranked third in the OECD countries for obesity prevalence. The United States also rated very highly in physical activity, at around 60%. That was twice as high as Japanese respondents, yet the rate of obesity in the two countries is reversed.[18]

Whether the value of exercise is in burning up calories or switching off physiological drivers of the metabolic syndrome, it's clear that on the whole we don't do enough physical activity. Educating or persuading people to engage in recreational activity is largely ineffective. Large-scale sporting events such as the Olympics or the World Cup don't seem to inspire individuals to become more active either. American football fans reported gaining between 20 and 45 pounds per season—presumably as a result of eating and drinking while glued to the sofa and the television set. Non-discretionary energy expenditure associated with work seems to offer the greatest opportunities for exercise. Cities that encourage walking and cycling and have efficient public transport systems are associated with active transport to and from work.[19]

Exercise is good for us and I'm a fan of any initiative that makes it easier for us to do more of it. But experience with my overweight patients has taught me that it's not practical to suggest exercise for weight loss. Mostly because people are unable to substantially change their behavior and sometimes because exercise makes them hungry and they eat more to compensate. Until our cities are rebuilt and public transport made more attractive we need other solutions. Can the pharmaceutical industry help us out?

3

Can drugs or surgery make us thin?

As a newly qualified endocrinologist in the early 1990s, I anticipated treating obesity as we do hypertension—with a combination of medications with different mechanisms of action. In the era of designer drugs, producing medicines to alter appetite, and perhaps metabolism, seemed quite plausible. Of course the prevalence of obesity at that time was quite small, perhaps equivalent to heart disease now, so a conventional medical approach to the problem made sense. As with heart disease, a small proportion of those affected needed more than medication and might require surgery instead.

But the trickle of patients has turned into a tsunami. Doctors continue to prescribe diets, though they are usually hopeless for anything other than short-term weight loss. The solutions for the populace lie in our environment. But we still need effective treatment for the very overweight who suffer with illness and disability that could be relieved by weight loss. Can we look to the pharmaceutical industry or to surgeons for assistance with this group at least?

Do any medicines work?

Although global obesity is a relatively new phenomenon people have made money out of putative cures for obesity for centuries. Tape worms, raspberry ketones, green coffee bean extract, an extract from the African moringa tree, and Korean pine nuts have all been peddled. Thehealthsite.com suggests that soaking the lentil known as 'horse gram' overnight and drinking the filtered concoction will cure obesity. Apparently this is popular in Ayurvedic medicine for the treatment of renal stones, piles, fluid retention, menstrual problems, colds, and diabetes. Meanwhile, drug companies have been working flat out for years on modern alternatives to this quackery. With a predicted market of 700 million obese people in 2015, who can blame them?

But so far, each new discovery has proved to be not so wonderful after all. In the 1930s, drug companies developed amphetamines as an alternative to ephedrine as a treatment for asthma. In 1937 an oral version called Benzedrine came on the market, promising to treat depression, narcolepsy, and even Parkinson's disease as well as suppressing appetite. The war accelerated its popularity; both the US and British armies supplied recruits with the drug (the German and Japanese armies used methamphetamine) to keep them awake during night missions. The beat poets immortalized Benzedrine (Benny) in the 1950s, and the 1966 bestselling novel *Valley of the*

Dolls described the lives of three women who were addicted to a combination of Benzedrine and barbiturates. Judy Garland took Benzedrine to control her weight until her death from a drug overdose at the age of 47. The drug continued to be used as speed until 1979, when it was banned after a number of 'diet pill' related deaths.

In the mid-1990s a combination of two 'non-speedy' amphetamine-type drugs called Dexfenfluramine was released as a modern appetite suppressant. This drug raises the chemical serotonin which acts in a number of ways including the control of mood (low levels are associated with depression), as well as altering the emptying rate of the stomach.[1] I can remember the marketing of Fen-phen, as it became known, and in particular the pharmaceutical company reassuring us that the possibility of valvular heart disease was low. Valvular heart disease had been identified as a rare but potentially fatal side effect of serotonin-raising drugs that had led to the withdrawal of older diet drugs. The trouble is that while drug companies are required to undertake research to pick up problems prior to a drug's release, these studies just aren't equipped to detect rare problems that may nonetheless be related to that drug. Sure enough, in 1996, after 18 million prescriptions had been filled, new cases of unexpected heart disease started to be reported by those prescribed Fen-phen.[2] While the incidence of these was still extremely low, the relative risk of developing the very serious complication of damaged heart valves was 20 times higher in those taking the medication than those who weren't, and the combination was withdrawn in 1997. For many years afterwards doctors were required to track down and submit anxious patients to echocardiograms to look for diseased heart valves.

Another drug that has come and gone is Rimonobant, which also acts in the brain and blocks the naturally occurring receptor for cannabis. Predictably this drug is quite good at suppressing appetite (no more munchies) but it's no surprise that it can also lower mood and in some individuals cause profound depression. This drug also has been withdrawn. Another agent, Sibutramine, was modestly effective at curbing hunger, but it had to go too because it caused an increase in heart rate and raised blood pressure, and as a result was likely to cause heart attacks and strokes.

Currently the most used medication is probably the anti-absorptive drug Orlistat, known to most as Xenical. This works by blocking the breakdown of fat in the gut. The drug isn't absorbed into the bloodstream but works directly in the gut and, apart from some very rare cases of liver injury, is free of dangerous side effects. Unfortunately, taking this medication with meals results in very oily bowel motions, and diarrhea and fecal incontinence are predictable consequences of eating fatty food. Some patients reported that this was a marvelous way of identifying the foods they shouldn't eat, but most people learned to simply skip the tablet when they planned to eat rich food. Others reported examples of catastrophic diarrhea when they had inadvertently eaten food that was fatty. The risk of incontinence, combined with considerable cost, has greatly limited its use.

There are diabetes drugs that reduce appetite as a side effect of their intended mechanism of lowering blood sugar levels. The oldest and best known of these is Metformin. Some patients can't take this medicine because it causes some nausea and diarrhea when you first start it. Diabetologists love it because it's one glucose-lowering agent that doesn't have weight gain as a side effect. Diabetes wastes calories because sugar builds up in the blood and spills out into the urine. This is corrected with medicines that drive glucose into the cells, and in addition people taking insulin often have to eat in order to prevent excessively low blood sugar at some times of the day. Occasionally patients taking Metformin actually lose weight and studies show that this is due to a reduction in calorie intake (because of feeling vaguely nauseated).

A few decades ago endocrinologists realised that Metformin could be useful in treating the cousin of type 2 diabetes—polycystic ovarian syndrome (PCOS). This condition results in reduced fertility in some overweight women with insulin resistance. Insulin resistance affects the way the ovaries respond to hormonal stimulation by the hypothalamus. Many of these women go on to develop type 2 diabetes later in life so it made sense to treat them with Metformin to see if it improved fertility. The good news is that it does, so the drug has now become routine treatment for PCOS, even in women with perfectly normal glucose levels. It is a small step to then prescribe Metformin for weight loss alone in people without diabetes or fertility problems. The problem is that it doesn't work very well, and people feel sick and/or get diarrhea at the doses required to have a significant effect on appetite. However, it is used for weight loss in non-diabetic patients who need to take modern anti-psychotic treatments which all have appetite stimulation as an unfortunate side effect.

Metformin is a very old drug and its modern equivalent is a designer drug developed from, believe it or not, the saliva of the gila monster. This South American lizard secretes a poisonous substance in its saliva that in humans results in profound appetite suppression—and, you guessed it, nausea. (The gila lizard is lucky that the saliva itself is no use as it is almost immediately broken down by enzymes in the bloodstream of humans.) Scientists have managed to reproduce the compound using gene technology and altered it so that as long as it is given by an injection under the skin, it lasts a whole day. Like Metformin, this class of drugs— called glucagon-like peptide-1 agonists (GLP-1 agonists)—was developed to treat type 2 diabetes (for which they are funded in the United States) but there are many trials under way to investigate their usefulness as weight loss drugs. Studies published so far suggest a modest weight loss of around 5–6% when used in trial conditions with support from dieticians.[3] As with other hormones these compounds need to lock in to a receptor on the surface of the cell in order to work and a related set of drugs which blocks that receptor has also been developed. In New Zealand at the time of writing these latter two drugs are not funded through Pharmac because of their considerable cost but many patients who can afford to buy them experience significant weight loss and improvements in their diabetes control as a result. The US Food and Drug Administration (FDA) is now looking at listing the GLP-1 agonists for weight loss alone.

What about medication to increase metabolism? The naturally occurring hormone thyroxine has a direct effect on metabolism, and when people develop an overactive thyroid gland due to the relatively common condition of Graves disease (named after the Dublin physician Sir Robert Graves) they usually lose weight as a result of the increase in metabolism. This is the opposite of Oprah's problem of *hypo*-thyroidism. Weight loss isn't invariable though, and I have seen overweight individuals gain weight when thyrotoxic because they so acutely sense the need for increased energy that they not only eat but overeat. Because thyroxine is a commonly prescribed medication for those with underactive thyroid glands, it has also been used to assist with weight loss. Unfortunately, the reason why treatment of an overactive thyroid gland is so important is that even modest elevations in thyroid hormone levels are toxic to heart muscle, resulting in a greatly increased risk of the fast, irregular heart rhythm called atrial fibrillation and, in extreme cases, of heart failure. Osteoporosis is also accelerated. Using tablets to boost thyroid hormone to levels higher than the normal range is equally dangerous.

While more drugs targeting different aspects of hunger are being developed all the time it's clear my prediction that obesity would be managed by medication is never going to be realized. The drugs have too many side effects and no government can afford to medicate most of the population.

Is surgery better?

Sooner or later most people realize their best efforts to lose weight using diets, exercise regimes, and sometimes drugs have failed to make a significant difference to their body size. The options are to give up or, ideally, to maximize health in other ways, ignoring weight. If you eat nutritious food, do as much exercise as you can, don't smoke, and treat the complications of obesity you will maintain good health. But for those with morbid obesity, and for some with less severe obesity and type 2 diabetes, bariatric surgery is sometimes recommended.

In 1954 a surgeon by the name of Kremen performed the first experimental bariatric operation—the jejuno-ileal bypass.[4] He divided the small intestine and joined it up again so it was reduced to around 10% of its original length. Most nutrient absorption occurs in the small gut, so this operation produces an immediate reduction in calories absorbed, irrespective of what is actually eaten. The leftover segment of small bowel wasn't removed in case the procedure needed to be reversed at some stage (many were), but was left attached as a 'blind loop' with the lower end joined up again to the large bowel. This surgical procedure was modified in the 1960s and again in the 1970s and some 10,000 people underwent a version of the operation.

Unfortunately this particular bypass procedure caused a lot of problems and some fatalities. Some people experienced dramatic weight loss, but as well as decreasing fat absorption they lost the ability to absorb fat-soluble vitamins, particularly vitamin D, leading to osteoporosis or even rickets. Many experienced bloating and diarrhea (5 to 14 times a day) from the unabsorbed fat and other nutrients as well as from an overgrowth of bacteria in the blind loop of the intestine. About 5% of people developed some degree of liver failure. In 1974 a report from surgical centers on their experience with these operations identified an unexpected problem of kidney stones. This affected 10% of the patients with the removal of at least one kidney. There were three deaths in the 52 patients including one who, 12 months after surgery, died of a cardiac arrest from very low potassium levels as a result of diarrhea.[5]

By the late 1970s the reputation of bariatric surgery was very poor. A review article from 1981 quotes Payne (one of the early pioneers in the field):

[F]rom an ethical and moral aspect, all of these operations, gastric partitioning, gastric bypass and jejuno-ileal bypass, are being abused.

Too many operations are being done on patients who are not viable candidates and by surgeons who are not qualified or have no efficient follow-up programme. The malignant abuse of these operations will result in the surgical discreditation of the surgical approach to morbid obesity. This could result in the abandonment of the only practical method, at this time, for the treatment of the morbidly obese patient.[6]

In an effort to avoid surgery some patients opted for jaw-wiring instead. While a diet of milk or soup with vitamin supplements is highly effective, it sounds ghastly. Most people couldn't tolerate the splints, there was a risk of drowning if you vomited, and of course the weight was regained when the splints came off.

The Roux-en-Y gastric bypass has replaced the jejuno-ileal bypass. This operation severely restricts the size of the stomach in combination with a modest reduction in the length of the small bowel. In this procedure it's the stomach not the small bowel which ends up 10% of the original volume and this is combined with narrowing of the gastric outlet so that the tiny stomach empties slowly. The full stomach suppresses appetite so even patients who have dramatic weight loss rarely report hunger. In the early versions the fundus (top segment) was cut off from the rest to make a small stomach but unfortunately this tissue is expandable and when the remnant stomach stretched people who lost weight initially started to reaccumulate it. The operation was changed to a vertical staple line through the more rigid region of the stomach but even then some operations failed because the staples popped when the stomach stretched. In later operations a permanent separation was made by cutting right through the stomach and oversewing the incision. Surgeons experimented with the size of the gastric outlet—a larger opening actually allows people to eat a wider range of healthy food including vegetables. A tight outlet caused too much regurgitation so some people found themselves resorting to chocolate milkshakes for nourishment—and put on weight as a result. All of the original procedures were 'open' operations but most are now performed using a laparoscope through a keyhole incision.

An alternative to a bypass procedure is the laparoscopic adjustable gastric band (LAGB) which simply restricts the size of the stomach. In a relatively simple operation an inflatable band is placed around the stomach using a laparoscope and once everything is healed the band is inflated. This is done in a step-wise fashion over several weeks in order to achieve the maximum tolerable constriction. An advantage of the band is avoiding the problems of malabsorption that occur with bypassing the small bowel but that means weight loss isn't as reliable. Patients need follow-up appointments to ensure the band is inflated at the correct intervals and they have to stick to a low calorie diet. While the procedure is reversible, critics of the LAGB say the band often slips and causes problems requiring re-operation. For some, however, it is an effective treatment and it is certainly less expensive, making it a first choice for many people. Some of these patients later go on to a bypass procedure.

Bariatric procedures are now 60 years old and they continue to evolve. But which is the safest and most effective? In July 2013 the National Bariatric Surgical Registry in the United Kingdom reported on just under 80% of the surgeons and operations performed in the UK over the previous year. They found that even though patients on the whole were very obese with an average weight of about 310 pounds and had 3.6 additional medical problems, such as diabetes, sleep apnea, and hypertension, the procedures were very safe. The in-hospital mortality was only 0.07%, equivalent to a survival rate of 99.93%, and the average length of stay was very short at only 2.5 days.[7]

The best long-term efficacy and safety data comes from the Swedish Obese Subjects (SOS) study which is unique in being controlled, prospective, and long term. The subjects are 2,010 obese people who underwent gastric bypass (13%), gastric banding (19%), and vertical banded gastroplasty, stomach stapling without bypass of the small intestine (68%), compared with age- and weight-matched people who weren't offered surgery. At 20 years the average weight loss for the surgical group was –18% compared to –1% for the non-surgical group. The surgical group also had a reduction in mortality (71%) and a similar reduction in myocardial infarction (heart attacks), stroke, and in women, a decrease in cancer to 58% of the non-operative group. The really marked reduction though was in diabetes, with only 17 cases of diabetes in the surgical group for every 100 in the non-surgical group. Interestingly diabetes disappears almost immediately following bypass surgery—even before weight loss.[8]

What about surgery as treatment of diabetes?

In 2012 two studies were published side by side in the *New England Journal of Medicine*. The first article compared bariatric surgery with intensive medical therapy in obese patients with type 2 diabetes. The group had very high blood sugar levels and the primary endpoint was good diabetic control which they defined as a near normal HbA1c (glycosylated haemoglobin). Haemoglobin (Hb) is designed to carry oxygen around in the blood but it will also pick up glucose. The higher the glucose levels the more likely the Hb molecule will have a glucose stuck to it (glycosylation). This can be measured and is used routinely in clinic to assess the level of control over the preceding six weeks or so. The intensive medical therapy offered was as good as anyone could get with counseling, the latest diabetic drugs, and three monthly visits with a specialist at the prestigious Cleveland Clinic. The surgical group had either a Roux-en-Y gastric bypass or a sleeve gastrectomy. (The latter operation is a more simple version of the vertical banded gastroplasty with a reduction in stomach size but no bypass.) All patients improved their diabetes control at 12 months but only 12% of the medical group achieved the HbA1c goal compared to 42% in the gastric bypass group and 37% in the sleeve gastrectomy group. To get this improvement 38% of the medical group, but only 4% of the gastric bypass patients and 8% of the sleeve gastrectomy patients, had to use insulin. At the end of the study the medically treated group were on more medicines than at the start and the surgical group were on fewer.[9]

The next paper sounds the same but this group weighed more with a minimum BMI of 35 and their diabetes wasn't as badly controlled at the outset. They compared medical therapy to gastric bypass or a bilio-pancreatic diversion procedure (a bypass procedure without reducing the size of the stomach). At two years all of the medically treated patients still had diabetes but it had remitted in 75% of the gastric bypass group and 95% of the bilio-pancreatic diversion group.[10]

Both studies showed that with the bypass procedures diabetes control improved *immediately* following surgery (the next day) before any weight loss. This is due to changes in hormones secreted by the gut and less fat reaching the liver from the small bowel. These changes don't happen with gastric banding so bypass procedures are better for people with type 2 diabetes. For those with severe obesity, and perhaps with less severe obesity and type 2 diabetes, bariatric surgery is effective. It's a safe operation and for some people it's life saving. But while many of the early complications associated with malabsorption have been addressed there are significant side effects with this radical procedure. A bariatric surgical colleague said to me once that people undergoing this operation need to understand that they can never eat normally again.

Drugs mostly don't work. These expensive operations do. But they can never be the solution to the obesity epidemic because the numbers affected are vast. Preventative measures are our only hope of turning this epidemic around. But before deciding what these measures should be it's important to understand why it is that not everyone is fat. Genetics play a critical role in determining how we respond to our environment. Obesity is a classic example of geno-environmental interaction.

4

Is fatness inherited?

Toomaths are small people. Five generations back a Toomath settled in New Zealand to escape the Irish potato famine. We've been well nourished since then but only very gradually are we growing in height. When I meet my Toomath cousins at weddings and funerals I'm impressed at how strongly the smallness runs in our family. My daughters are slim; it's in their genes. I've been looking at the *Te Awamutu Courier* online— particularly at the photos of school kids. They look happy and healthy, but many more are overweight than when I attended Te Awamutu Primary School in the 1960s. It's the environment these children are growing up in, and particularly what they are eating, that's made the difference. But perhaps the genes they have inherited explain why most are getting fatter but some aren't.

Genes and body size

Today, scientists work on genetics using the most sophisticated laboratory technology. But the science of genes developed from observing the world around us. Gregor Mendel first uncovered the patterns of inheritance by experimenting on garden peas. Similarly, simple observation leads us to conclude that obesity is a genetically determined condition.

One indication of the genetic basis of obesity is the difference in the prevalence of obesity between people of one ethnicity and another in the same environment, and the effect of admixture when individuals from these different races have children. This is seen in Hawai'i where Hawaiian-Latino people are fatter than Hawaiians whereas Hawaiian-Asian people are slimmer.[1] Another is the fact that as obesity has become more common, the entire population hasn't become fatter. Instead, the usual bell-shaped distribution curve is skewed. People at the heavy end of the scale have become even fatter while there has been little shift in the weights of people at the lower end of the curve. This tells us that the environmental effect is uneven, and the skew can be explained by the differing genetic predisposition of individuals to gain weight.

Epidemiology is the study of diseases in populations, looking for patterns that might reveal causes. Using this science, epidemiologists see strong support for a genetic basis for obesity in the study of twins. Identical twins share all of their genes whereas non-identical or fraternal twins are just like siblings, with roughly half of the genes shared. This doesn't mean that identical twins will express their genes in exactly the same way because genetic conditions vary in their 'penetrance,' which is the likelihood

49

that a genetic message will be translated into physical reality. Predisposition to type 1 diabetes, for example, is actually more of a genetic disorder than type 2 diabetes. But most people with the predisposition don't go on to get the disease (it has low penetrance) so it is relatively rare, and most often there is only one family member with type 1 diabetes. But the key is that if a condition is genetically determined it should be seen in both identical twins much more often than it is seen in both fraternal twins. In the case of type 1 diabetes the twin pattern holds true. You have a 10% chance of developing type 1 diabetes if your *non*-identical twin has the problem but a 35% chance if you are an identical twin. Comparing the rates with which identical and non-identical twin pairs inherit a particular trait also allows you to separate out the influence of shared environment.

In 1986 the psychiatrist Albert Stunkard first examined the relative effects of genetics and rearing environments using the Danish adoption registry. The purpose of the registry was to study genetic influence in schizophrenia but he used the data collected to study the effect of adoption on body weight. He found almost no correlation between the weight of adopted children (now adults) and their adoptive parents despite the shared environment. Fortunately, the registry had recorded the weights and heights of the biological parents at the time of adoption and Stunkard discovered a close relationship between the weights of children and their biological parents. Eighty percent of those who had two obese biological parents were also obese—it was as if the rearing environment had no effect at all.[2]

Stunkard followed up this study by drawing on BMI information from a Swedish registry that included 25,000 same-sex twins born between 1886 and 1959. In this group were 311 twin pairs who were reared apart over several decades. (The twins had been separated as a result of economic hardship and/or death of the parents.) Almost half of the twins were separated in the first year of life and 82% by the time they were five. At the time of the study the twins were 58 years old on average. Once again, Stunkard found that the weights of the adopted family members were unrelated to the families who raised them, but the weights of the adult twins were closely matched, and it didn't matter whether the twins were separated early in life (before the age of 2) or later. This relationship was stronger for identical than fraternal twins. Mathematical modelling led Stunkard to conclude that weight was about 70% genetically determined.[3] The correlation wasn't restricted to obese people but held true across the complete range of body size. So, contrary to what most people believe, this evidence suggests that childhood environment has very little effect on adult weight.

There have in fact been many studies demonstrating the powerful effect of genetics on body size. A paper published in the journal *Behavior Genetics* in 1997 should have been the end of any speculation. The authors performed a meta-analysis of twin studies, family studies, and adoption studies that encompassed data from 25,000 twin pairs and 50,000 other family members. They used something called a structural equation model (Stealth) and showed matched weights in 74% of identical twins, 32% of non-identical twins and 25% of other siblings. They concluded 'genetic factors play a significant role in the causes of individual differences in relative body weight and human adiposity [obesity].'[4]

BMI is weight in kilograms divided by the square of the height in meters and is the usual measure of fatness across population studies, but it's only a surrogate measure for what really causes the metabolic problems of obesity. Diabetes, high cholesterol, hypertension, and fatty liver are related to the amount of fat around the internal organs within the abdominal cavity. The best measure of abdominal fatness is waist circumference but it's not often used in studies because it's hard to know exactly where your waist is and the measurement varies if you hold your stomach in or out. It's also a lot more intrusive than asking someone to stand on a set of scales. In children, waist circumference is increasing at an even faster rate than BMI. Professor Jane Wardle is a London psychologist with a special interest in eating behaviors of children and she looked at whether the genetic relationship holds true for this measure in the same way that it does for BMI. Her study of 5092 UK twin pairs between 8 and 11 years of age shows heritability accounts for about 70% of the variability for both BMI and waist circumference but there isn't complete overlap. For 60% of the children the waist circumference and weight went up in parallel but 40% were either fat around the middle but otherwise skinny or vice versa. So it appears you can separately inherit a tendency to fatness and a tendency to accumulating fat around the middle.[5]

Such close studies of various forms of fatness are interesting. They hint at why there is racial variation in the susceptibility to type 2 diabetes and other metabolic problems. At any BMI Asian people are more likely to accumulate fat in the abdomen than Europeans who in turn are fatter around the middle than Pacific Islanders. The cut-off values for a healthy BMI have been adjusted to account for this being 23, 25 and 27 respectively. Acquiring fat around the middle is a normal part of ageing and is one reason we are more likely to become diabetic as we get older.

The hunt for the fat genes

Knowing that our genotype (genetic pattern) has a powerful impact on our weight is one thing, identifying the specific genes responsible is another.

One way to make sense of the ways in which genes can produce disease is to examine the rare but pure examples of monogenic disorders, where a single gene defect is enough to cause disease, for instance cystic fibrosis. These examples help us to understand the underlying biological problem (the pathogenesis) and from this we may be able to extrapolate to the more common polygenic disorders, of which obesity is a classic example, where very many genes determine the outcome or phenotype. Animal models are also helpful because they provide us with the opportunity to breed entire populations with a known genotype and to study the effects of this.

The best example of a gene variant causing obesity is provided by the ob/ob mouse. This strain of mouse, identified in 1950, has a genetic mutation on chromosome 6 and a voracious appetite.[6] As a consequence the mouse becomes extremely fat (on average, three times the weight of a normal mouse). Researchers in 1973 transfused these mice with blood from normal mice and they immediately stopped their frantic eating and their weight normalised, indicating that the chromosome abnormality caused a failure of satiety (food satisfaction) which was corrected by something in the bloodstream of a normal mouse.[7] This had to be a hormone. Hormones float around in the bloodstream but have very specific effects because they need to lock in to a receptor in order to work. These receptors are only found in certain tissues and become activated when the hormone attaches to them.

The db/db mouse is a different mouse strain with a predisposition to diabetes, and researchers determined that these mice must have a genetic defect in the *receptor* for leptin because although they were physically identical to the ob/ob mice, the abnormality didn't correct with blood from normal mice.

Finally, in 1994, after eight years of research, the geneticist Jeffrey Friedman made a replica of (cloned) the ob gene and showed that it did indeed encode the appetite-suppressing hormone that was missing from the mutant ob/ob mice.[8] He called this hormone leptin—after the Greek word *leptos*, meaning thin. Friedman's group then used recombinant DNA technology to produce the leptin hormone. This technique, developed in 1972 and first used to make insulin, is when the DNA that codes for human insulin is inserted into yeast DNA. When the yeast is stimulated to grow it produces the hormone insulin. They then conducted the defining experiment of injecting leptin into the abdomen of the ob/ob mouse twice a day. This switched off the excessive appetite and the mice lost weight and their fat mass fell from 12.2% to 7%.[9]

This news was greeted with great excitement. Immediately the hunt was on for the same gene abnormality in humans. It does exist, but it's very rare. Several Pakistani families and at least one Turkish family have been identified with homozygous mutations (carrying two copies of the variant gene) causing leptin deficiency. Once again severe obesity is caused by exaggerated appetite and the children of these families show a good response to leptin injections, with appetite switching off and a return to normal body weight.[10] But unfortunately in most obese people leptin levels are high because the hormone comes from fat cells. There is the lingering thought that perhaps obese people have a *relative* leptin deficiency, and that the levels should really be higher than they are for someone of that weight, and if they were, then appetite would be suppressed. The evidence for this, however, is weak. Obese people have been given leptin injections experimentally but they have not lost weight.

Another, more common single gene defect leading to pathological obesity in humans is Prader-Willi syndrome. This affects about one person in 15,000 and, like leptin-deficient individuals, people with Prader-Willi syndrome feel as though they are starving and food-seeking behaviors are exaggerated. Parents of these children lock the pantry and put bolts on the refrigerator and still the affected person is invariably obese.

What these two monogenic (and other) examples tell us is that variation from one person to another with regard to body size is much more likely to be a matter of altered appetite than altered metabolism. But we also know that in the vast majority of cases, obesity is not the result of a single gene defect. It is a polygenetic condition and isn't even necessarily an abnormality; the gene variations are those that conferred a survival advantage in times of famine. Now that insufficient calorie intake is a rare phenomenon, those who have inherited many of the gene variations favoring food-seeking behaviors are more likely to become obese, those with a few of these variants may be overweight, and those with none may well remain slim, despite the obesity-promoting environment in which we all live. Identifying these other behavior-modifying genes is the next quest.

'Normal' obesity

The obvious place to start looking for genes is with people who demonstrate the phenotype, or physical manifestation of obesity, then look for the genotype, or underlying genes. Finding obesity-promoting genes can be done in one of two ways. The first is by taking genes thought likely to be associated with obesity, those associated with insulin or leptin for example, and studying the genetic material to see which variations are more common in obese people when compared to thin. This is known as the candidate gene approach. Sadaf Farooqi, Stephen O'Rahilly, and their group at Cambridge University, who lead the Genetics of Obesity Study, use this technique when studying unusually obese children. For example, the compound melanocortin is found in the appetite center of the brain and is needed for leptin to work. When they went looking they found variations in the gene which codes for the melanocortin (MCR4) receptor and that having the obesity-promoting version of the gene accounts for between 1% and 6% of early onset obesity.[11]

The human genome project which started in 1995 has provided an alternative way to go 'hunting for genes.' This project, costing US$200 million a year, was an incredible example of international collaboration and saw the scientific community cooperating to map out the genetic sequence of human DNA. Since its completion, geneticists have used genome wide associated scanning (GWAS) to look for genes which show up more often than expected in the population of interest—in this case, obese people. Scanning in this way allows researchers to detect genes not normally associated with obesity. The best example of success with this approach was finding the fat mass and obesity (FTO) gene, hitherto unsuspected of having any role in human metabolism but which in fact accounts for a significant amount of the genetic variability among obese people. Of a large group of adults who were studied, 16% were homozygous and on average they weighed about 6 pounds more than the adults who didn't carry a copy of the at-risk gene.[12]

In May 2014 the *New England Journal of Medicine* published an important paper describing a mutation that causes the metabolic syndrome—susceptibility to weight gain, high blood pressure, heart disease, and fatty liver. In a population in West Iran where leanness is the norm, some members of three families developed these problems at an early age. This didn't occur randomly within families; the pattern was one of autosomal dominance, which is where you have two copies of the gene—one from each parent—but the metabolic-syndrome-promoting gene takes precedence. This is the same dominance seen with eye color where an individual ends up with brown eyes irrespective of whether they have two brown eye genes, or one brown and one blue (while only those who inherit two blue eye genes end up with blue eyes). Knowing that these problems had to be genetic, the authors went hunting for a mutation and found the same genetic abnormality in all of the affected members from three separate families. It wasn't found in any of the slim family members.[13] While this particular abnormality is rare the discovery is important because it will provide clues as to why so many of the population develop these problems when offered excess calories.

By early 2015 a total of 97 genetic variations like the FTO gene had been identified as having a significant relationship to obesity.[14] But each variation by itself accounts for only a small proportion of what is known to be genetic control of body size.

So researchers are now trying to understand the additive effects of these single gene variations.[15] If you are unlucky enough to inherit several of these energy-seeking or -storing genes you are more likely to become obese in the current environment than someone who has only a few. On the other hand, you are probably going to be the person who will do best if marooned on a desert island. At this stage, though, the gene abnormalities identified account for less than 5% of the variance in BMI.[16]

Our genes do make us fat. But we can't change our genes to make us slim.

Does obesity start in the womb?

Do we describe what happens in the womb as genetic or environmental? It seems like it could be both. Exposure to certain conditions in the womb can have effects that persist throughout a person's life. Both under- and over-nutrition, for example, increase the likelihood that a person will develop obesity, type 2 diabetes, and heart disease—independent of any familial tendency.

The best example of the effect of under-nutrition comes from a study of the children born to mothers who survived the Dutch famine. Towards the end of the Second World War a failed attempt by the Allied forces to capture a bridge giving access to Dutch farmlands led to the relative starvation of the population in the west of the Netherlands. In December 1943 rations for adults in Amsterdam consisted of 1,800 kilocalories per day, in October the following year this was down to 1,400 kilocalories and between December 1944 and April 1945 the rations were between 400 and 800 kilocalories.[17] Compare this to the kilocalorie requirement of around 2,000 per day for a young, slim, relatively sedentary woman. The Dutch supplemented the rations with black-market supplies and locally grown food to some extent but there was significant starvation. Approximately 20 years later, the Dutch weighed 300,000 military recruits and matched them with their mothers' birth records. Using birth date the researchers determined whether the mother had been exposed to famine while pregnant, and whether this was in the first, middle, or last trimester of pregnancy. What they found was that under-nutrition during the first half of pregnancy resulted in 19-year-olds who were significantly more likely to be obese and researchers concluded that this was the result of some sort of programming of the hypothalamus to increase appetite. However, under-nutrition later in the pregnancy produced thin babies and thinner adults and the theory was that starvation at this critical stage resulted in a smaller than normal number of fat cells.[18]

The more relevant question today is whether obesity begets obesity as a result of maternal *over*-nutrition. Studies show that mothers who are obese or who have higher than normal blood sugar levels during pregnancy may *overfeed* the baby. The fetus responds to the higher than normal sugar levels in the placental blood supply by increasing insulin from its own pancreas and this drives fat storage in the baby. The overfed baby can be a problem in itself. Very big babies are hard to deliver, usually requiring caesarean section, and the ramped-up insulin production predisposes the baby to hypoglycemia (low blood sugar) during the first couple of days before a mother's milk comes in. But the real concern is whether such intra-uterine exposure can lead to adult obesity over and above what would be expected from parental genes and the rearing environment. Observing Pima Indian children indicates that this is the case. These people were thin in their original mountainous environment but now most live on reservations in Arizona and have an extremely high rate of obesity and type 2 diabetes. If a Pima Indian child is born to a mother after she develops diabetes, he or she has a higher likelihood of being obese as a teenager than a sibling born to the same mother before she develops diabetes.[19] The reverse also holds true. Obese women who undergo bariatric surgery give birth to smaller babies who go on to have a lower rate of obesity when compared to their siblings born before the mother loses weight.[20]

It's not too surprising that the environment during fetal development can have effects that last a person's whole lifetime, but there is evidence now that the effect can be passed on to the next generation too. For this to occur, the genome must be altered. This happens all the time as a result of random mutations but it can also happen as a result of additional molecules (such as a methyl group) sticking on to the protein of DNA in a way that switches genes on or off. The term used to describe this is 'epigenetics.' In 2009, more than 40 years after the publication of the observational study of survivors of the Dutch famine, geneticists reported that there are indeed differences in the DNA methylation (methyl attached to the DNA) of the offspring depending on when during the pregnancy the mother was starved. This supports the theory that in addition to reprogramming the appetite center, uterine conditions close to the time of conception also cause genetic changes that alter the risk of becoming obese, not only for the baby but for the baby's children.[21]

From genotype to phenotype

Having established a genetic basis for obesity, and additionally identified some of the genes responsible, the next question to be answered is how do genetics influence body size? In other words, how do we get from the genotype to the phenotype? If you asked most people on the street, including those who are overweight, they would probably say that genes determine whether you have a fast or slow metabolism. But we know that the rate at which you burn energy, the metabolic rate, actually goes up with increasing weight because it takes more energy to drive a bigger body. Most genetic variations associated with obesity identified so far have caused an increase in appetite.

Human beings become overweight simply because they consume more food than required for a given level of energy expenditure. If we agree that this behaviour is genetically mediated then we need also to assume that in ethnic groups where obesity is more prevalent, there is a clustering of these genotypes. One theory that has been around for a long time is that of the thrifty genotype. This term was coined by epidemiologists to explain the ethnic variability in the prevalence of type 2 diabetes. The explanation is that in people from hunter-gatherer cultures, efficient food storage is an adaptation to an intermittent food supply and when the food becomes continuous and abundant the result is obesity and type 2 diabetes. In cultures that have had a long history of a regular food supply this adaptation is not necessary.[22] At the time this theory was first proposed in the 1960s, the rate of obesity among Pacific people living in the islands was low when compared to those who had migrated to countries like New Zealand. Since then of course motorbikes and soft drinks

61

have arrived in the Pacific and obesity rates are as high there as in New Zealand.

Behaviors that result in the seeking out and consumption of high-energy foods must have been powerfully protective during times of famine. The genes which promote these behaviors would therefore have been selected for over the generations. If in recent times the food supply hasn't been secure this effect is likely to be greater. If there are additional selection pressures such as prizing 'largeness' as a physical characteristic then you can see how these genes may be more prevalent in one ethnic group or culture compared to another. It's possible we may now start to see biological selection pressure for genes promoting *slimness* because obesity is associated with relative infertility. There is also the potential effect of societal preference for slimness as a characteristic but this isn't entirely clear-cut. According to studies asking about preference, men are more likely to choose a slim partner over an overweight one, but for women physical characteristics aren't such an issue when selecting a partner. Needless to say, selection processes like this will change the population genetics over thousands of years not decades.

The case for the genetic control of appetite

Anyone who is a parent knows that so much of our child's behavior is innate—resistant to anything we might do to change it. Why are some kids reluctant eaters from birth while a sibling will 'eat like a horse'? And many of these behaviors persist. I have two friends, both very intelligent, fit, middle-aged women. One of them is large and eats very big meals with gusto. The other is very slim and although she likes food she usually won't clear her plate. (I'm somewhere in between.) The assumption is that this is conscious, or at least learned, but I think it's genetic. To work out whether the genetic determination of obesity is through variability in appetite researchers could try a few different tests. They could assess appetite in those with a known genotype. Or they could assume an obesity genotype in those who are overweight and see to what extent appetite tracks with this. Finally, they could look at twins again to see if eating behavior shows the predictable patterns between identical and fraternal twins.

Using the knowledge that carrying a certain variant of the FTO gene increases your chance of becoming obese, Professor Jane Wardle assessed a group of 3,337 children in the United Kingdom with the Child Eating Behaviour Questionnaire and also had them genotyped. Parents answered questions such as 'Would your child still eat lunch if he/she had a snack just before?' and 'How would your child respond to the offer of ice cream?' Parents know these things. My mother tells me that as a child, I was never too sick to eat, and as an adult, even working long hours as a trainee doctor, I don't think I ever missed a meal! As predicted, the children who were homozygous for the obesity version of the FTO gene were a whole lot hungrier than the other children.[23] Another study looked at appetite traits in Hispanic children and found correlations with another of the genotypes known to be associated with obesity (MCR4, the melanocortin receptor gene).

The second way to look at the correlation between genes and appetite is to assume an underlying genetic basis to body size and see to what extent measures of appetite change with weight. One such study looked at the eating behaviors (assessed by

63

the same Child Eating Behaviour Questionnaire) of 7–12-year-olds over the complete spectrum of body size from under- to overweight. They found that early satiety, slow eating, and food fussiness were all more common in the slimmer children and food responsiveness, enjoyment of food, emotional overeating, and desire to drink were all associated with those of heavier weights and these relationships were unaffected by age, sex, race, or parental education.[24] Just like my friends.

In the United Kingdom, parents of twins born between March and December 2007 were invited to join Gemini, a study designed by Professor Jane Wardle to look at the effects of environment on weight and development up until the age of five years. Wardle asked the parents of these 4,804 infants to answer a survey and found that appetite variability is obvious from an early age, no surprise to most mothers, and that it shows the pattern of genetic inheritance. The appetite questions rated the babies' enjoyment of food, the speed with which they drank, whether they became full easily, and so forth. The questionnaire refers to *food* and to *eating*, but these were three-month-old babies and the food was breast milk. All of the measures of appetite were higher in the heavier babies. The evidence for these behaviors being genetic is that the appetite scores were much closer for the identical twins than they were for non-identical twins.[25] This really supports Albert Stunkard's adopted twin studies which suggest that the variation between individuals has nothing to do with the environment and is all about genes.

Taste and psychology also play a role in appetite, and they too seem to be genetic. For example, certain foods taste differently depending on your genes. Only some people taste the compound propylthiouracil as bitter and a study which divided up those who could and could not taste the compound went on to look at preferences for other foods and found that the non-tasters were more tolerant of both bitter foods and foods with a high fat content. Emotional eating and food addiction play more of a role with some people than with others and, just as with alcohol, genetic susceptibility is likely. Addictive personality traits can be determined using tools to assess sensitivity to reward and researchers have found that these traits are associated with a tendency to emotional overeating.

Fidgeting, brown fat, and gut bacteria

Body size is a matter of energy in versus energy out and so far most of the discussion with regard to genetic determinants of body size has been about energy in. On the energy-out side of the equation are the experiments where individuals given identical amounts of food over and above their energy requirements gain weight to a variable degree and this has loosely been attributed to changes in 'metabolism.' Researchers conducted early experiments with volunteer inmates from Vermont Prison, first overfeeding the prisoners, then underfeeding them (to return to baseline). The aim was to identify the cellular and hormonal changes associated with weight gain. From these experiments they learned that fat cells don't change in number, they just enlarge and shrink with weight gain and loss.[26] Researchers observed that the men varied in the amount of weight that they gained despite matched food intake and most had difficulty keeping the extra weight on. The exceptions were a couple of men who, it transpired, had a family history of obesity.

There are a number of explanations for variations in the energy-out side of the equation but studies have shown that there really isn't much variation in basal metabolic rate or in postprandial thermogenesis, the energy burned up by the act of eating. When we overeat we increase our energy expenditure (there are *some* homeostatic mechanisms favoring slimness) due to non-exercise activity thermogenesis, which describes behavior such as fidgeting, changing posture, and so forth.[27] While this is only a small component of the energy-out side of the equation, it seems to be familial and may be another reason for variation in susceptibility to weight gain.

Mammals generate heat either by shivering or by a process called thermogenesis, from burning stores of brown fat. The latter process is important in animals but brown fat isn't thought to have a role in humans because it's not usually seen except in newborn babies. Recently though it's been identified in adults on PET (positron emission tomography) scans and the thought is that slim people may burn off extra energy in this tissue. The process is described as 'uncoupled' metabolism and is akin to cycling fast on a bicycle that's slipped out of gear. Support for this idea comes from finding brown fat in a series of young women with constitutional leanness (lucky them).[28]

And I wonder whether we'll find variations in mitochondrial function making it easier for some people to exercise compared to others. There are rare genetic disorders of mitochondria that result in fatigue and exercise intolerance and the suspicion is that these conditions are underdiagnosed.[29] In the meantime there is the role of our gut flora to consider.

Living in our gut are more than 100 trillion viruses and bacteria. I'm not exaggerating. This is 10 times the number of cells in the human body so perhaps humans are no more than bacteria support systems—like a giant agar plate. Not only is this population huge but it is relatively unstable and can be altered within 24 hours by a change in diet. Food that isn't digested in the stomach and small intestine (cellulose and other fibrous foods) reaches the large bowel where it either ferments or undergoes further digestion. Fermentation produces gas but it also induces gut cells to release the satiety hormones GLP-1 and ghrelin, which are absorbed in the bloodstream and act in the hypothalamus (the appetite control center of the brain) to make us feel full. Extra digestion on the other hand results in additional calorie extraction. The extent to which one or the other occurs depends on our 'microbiota.' This term is used to describe the make-up of the bacterial population in the gut in the same way we might describe the 'flora' of a forest. There are several large groupings of bacteria displaying different characteristics, with the furmicutes group favoring calorie extraction when compared to the bacteroidetes group. Support for an alteration in the gut microflora as a cause of obesity comes from the farming industry where apparently the use of probiotics (live organisms found in such foods as yogurt) and low-dose antibiotics is commonly practiced to induce weight gain in stock. Presumably the antibiotics kill off certain strains of bacteria and these are replaced with 'healthier' bacteria derived from probiotics. This works in pigs, ducks, calves, and chickens and experimentally in mice. Why not in humans?[30] There is also evidence that our diet influences what we grow in our gut. A high-fat diet is associated with increased numbers of the unhealthy organisms but also with leakiness of the gut lining. Bacteria leaking across the epithelium causes low-grade systemic inflammation which is associated with obesity, insulin resistance, and an increased risk of atherosclerosis, plaque build-up on arteries leading to stroke and heart attacks.[31]

Not only is the alteration of our bowel flora a possible contributor to obesity, but there is the tantalizing prospect of inducing slimness by manipulating our colonic population using prebiotics (dietary fiber) and probiotics. A study of mice, conducted with the aim of shifting the microbiota to reduce obesity, used a probiotic and the antibiotic Vancomycin. Only the antibiotic was effective. But as Vancomycin is one of those antibiotics doctors like to keep up their sleeve to treat serious infections the last thing anyone wants is to create resistance to this drug by using it as a weight loss agent. We'll have to do better than that.[32] Fecal transplants are being used to treat cases of resistant diarrhea and experiments are under way where feces from lean donors are inserted into obese people to see if lasting changes in the gut microbiome can be achieved.

It's one thing to identify a relationship between obesity and gut flora but another thing entirely to change the flora and expect the body shape or size to follow. What is emerging is that while both host genetics and the gut microbiome influence whether we are fat or thin, our genes may well determine what we grow in the gut.[33] In a study conducted to look at the effects of probiotics on allergy, researchers took fecal samples from a group of Finnish children from birth to the age of 7. When the 7-year-olds were divided up into overweight and obese and compared to a similar number of normal weight children, the study found those with higher numbers of the 'good' fecal bacteria at birth are more likely to be of normal weight at the age of 7.[34] My prediction is that we'll find the gut microbiota are dictated by genes *and* diet, and improving nutrition may well induce healthy bacteria but it will also reduce obesity. In other words, there may not be a causal relationship between the gut microbiota and obesity even if the two are linked.

What makes the difference between your weight and mine is our genes. At least two-thirds of the variability in BMI between us is due to genetic factors. And at least 40% of the variability in body size is due to variability in appetite.[35]

We are eating more and we are getting fatter. But our genes haven't changed. What's made the difference in the number of people who are overweight now compared to 30 years ago is our environment.

PART 2

Why our modern world makes us fat

5

How new ways of living have led to new ways of eating

While genes provide the best explanation for one person being thin and another being fat, they can't account for the increase in obesity over the last 30 years. Our genes have stayed the same but there has been a dramatic change in the world in which we live. Prior to the technological advances of the last century, work was strenuous and food was expensive. A worker needed to spend much of his income just to replace the calories expended on the job. If he didn't have a job, and lived in a country or time without a welfare system, starvation was a real possibility. Over the decades food has become cheaper to produce to the point where supply exceeds demand. At the same time work has become more sedentary. Today the worker must now *pay* to do physical activity, and not working, with welfare support to provide food, is more likely to result in obesity than starvation.[1]

Where we live changes what we eat

When I was growing up in Te Awamutu the population of the town was 6,000. I lived within walking distance of the primary school and local college and biking distance of the intermediate school. Although I wasn't any good at sports I played netball on Saturdays and later hockey. As primary school children we learned to swim in the tiny swimming pool and spent much of the summer hanging out at the town baths. We had television from the time I was 6 years old (never a color set) and the two channels were required to have two non-commercial days a week and a minimum of 30% local content. Car ownership was relatively high with one car for every 2.6 people and I sat for my driver's license when I was 15. Census data from 1976 when I was 21 tells us that people married young with 75% of brides being less than 24 and one in three less than 20—requiring parental consent.

But perhaps the biggest difference between now and then was the food we ate. New Zealanders spend a relatively high proportion of total household expenditure on food and this proportion hasn't changed between 1974 (17.6%) and 2013 (17.3%). But back in 1974 we spent a third more of that expenditure on fruit and vegetables and twice as much on meat, poultry and fish.[2] Milk was relatively cheaper at 4 cents for a bottle (delivered) because it was heavily subsidized. There were subsidies on bread and eggs too.

There was no supermarket and my memory of food being available outside normal working hours is that it was limited to what was sold at the gas station and a few dairies. In November 1975 a restaurant meal of steak and eggs cost NZ$2.39 and a hamburger was 45 cents. Takeaways came from the fish and chip shop and soft drinks were bought by your father in a wooden crate from the liquor store as a treat at Christmas. When I was a bit older I remember returning from holiday and stopping at a bakery in Huntly that sold hot bread on Sunday evenings. This was a huge novelty given that bread was otherwise delivered to the mailbox—along with the bottles of milk—with a strip of white paper around the middle. But by the time I was at intermediate school Coke and Fanta were well established, even if we didn't get to drink them very often, and I remember the first McDonald's opening in Porirua in 1976. Just prior to that, I had a taste of American-style fast food when I spent one summer working in a Big Tex restaurant at Paraparaumu. Chicken was precrumbed and fried and when a new order came in we would throw a piece into the pressurized deep-fryer for another blast. Rock-hard bread rolls became light and fluffy in a microwave—not seen domestically in New Zealand for another decade. The methods of cooking were so novel and outlandish it was almost worthwhile wearing cowgirl outfits to learn these fast food techniques; I still remember chucking frozen peas onto a hot plate and clamping a pot lid on top to create steam.

We adored everything American—especially that portrayed in Coca-Cola advertising. We were intrigued by what we saw on television of their convenience foods (milk in cartons!) but we were being taught to cook food from scratch in our lessons at intermediate school. Meat and three veg prevailed in the homes around New Zealand but my mother is an adventurous cook and I remember her bottling spaghetti with tomato sauce 'Italian style,' until one batch exploded in the pantry. There was one restaurant in the town—patronized on birthdays and anniversaries—so dinners were eaten at home, at the table. Hamburgers and milkshakes truly were occasional foods.

My experience of a small town upbringing wasn't unusual. Data, again from the census of 1976, tell us that only 45% of the population lived in cities of greater than 25,000 with 25% of the population living in the country or in towns with a population of 10,000 or less. By 2001, 80% of New Zealanders lived in urban areas of 30,000 or more. In the developed world migration from rural areas to the cities has been steady over the last century. In the developing world, though, the shift from rural to urban is recent and in some countries it coincides with large population increases. This is producing massive growth of up to 5% per year in the urban populations of Sub-Saharan Africa and Asia. Urbanization results in a higher participation of women in the workforce and, as a consequence, a move from time-consuming meal preparation to convenience food.[3]

Does urbanization lead to reduced physical activity? It depends on the type of urban development and its impact on leisure and transport. Access to recreational venues for physical leisure activity is often better in the city but the impact of transport can vary widely. New Zealanders like to live in suburbs and for most this means owning a car. A 2006 study found that 82% of New Zealanders owned a car, third ranked in the world after Saudi Arabia (86%) and the United Sates (90%). New Zealanders are one of the lowest users of public transport with only 5.6% getting to work this way, ranking us 22 out of 28 countries. On average, New Zealanders now spend 4.75 hours a week driving compared with four hours 20 years ago.[4] This is in contrast to cities like Amsterdam or Kyoto where cars are shunned in favour of bicycles, or New York where there is a high number of shops and venues in a small area so that walking is a realistic way of getting to them.

The density of the population living in the area is the most important factor contributing to increased physical activity, with a high number of retail and cultural destinations after that. Researchers looking for features of urban design that would serve as a proxy for walkability identified the number of complex traffic intersections as something that inversely correlates with obesity in the United States. Presumably these are more likely to be found in dense inner-city areas with slow-moving traffic.[5] But tools like this are pretty hopeless because they don't factor in the level of crime or the effects of highways or of large bodies of water that get in the way of where you are going. Now software developers have produced more sophisticated scoring tools for assessing the walkability of your particular neighbourhood, using information from Google Maps, census, and real estate data. Results are scored from 1 to 100 and using the Walk Score website I see the area around Auckland Hospital is rated at 75, which the site suggests is 'pretty walkable' and that 'residents in the area can probably manage without a car' (true).

In terms of change over time, it's a mixed picture. As we've seen, the time New Zealanders spend driving to work has increased by about a fifth in the past 20 years. The problem is worst in Auckland where the urban sprawl has been encouraged by transport policies which strongly favor cars.[6] Public transport use is low and only 3.5% of the population walks to work. For those who travel to work by car, 90% are single occupants.[7] This phenomenon is being replicated around the world with the most dramatic recent changes in low- and middle-income countries. Studies comparing car ownership worldwide find rich countries are relatively saturated,[8] but in India, Pakistan, and China the rate of car ownership is growing at approximately twice the rate of income increase.[9] In high-income countries, as people move back to the inner city, there are signs that car usage is falling in favor of public transport. Whereas I had my driving license at 15, one of my daughters obtained hers at the age of 24 and the 28-year-old cycles and takes the bus. Getting your license later is a trend in rich countries throughout the world. In Europe the share of young households without cars increased from 20% to 28% between 1998 and 2008 and Americans between the ages of 16 and 34 with incomes greater than $70,000 increased their public transport use by 100% between 2001 and 2009.[10]

Urban design and food consumption overlap most obviously when we look at the distribution of fast food outlets. While it is true that having shops within easy walking distance encourages physical activity, if those retail outlets are selling cheap, energy-dense food the sum effect is likely to be bad. The effect of proximity is particularly strong for people who access these venues on foot—adolescents and work-at-home mothers. Confirmation of this comes from a study in London, Ontario, where 800 children aged 11–13 were asked to report on the frequency with which they bought food from fast food outlets or convenience stores. Researchers correlated the data with the number of fast food outlets and convenience stores within 1 kilometer of both their home and school and, unsurprisingly, if one of these outlets was nearby the children were more likely to buy food from them.[11] The plot thickens when you look at proximity to fast food outlets and the ethnicity of the local population. In a study performed in 20 secondary schools in Minnesota, Black, Hispanic, and Native Americans were more likely to have fast food restaurants near where they lived than White and Asian

Americans, and adolescent males living near fast food outlets ate more junk food.[12]

Watching television makes us fat

It seems faintly ridiculous to single out one piece of technology and give it special status in the face of complex environmental changes, but TV does require attention. The steam engine and perhaps the car were similarly potent agents of change and access to the internet certainly exceeds these. A survey by Common Sense Media in 2013 found that 38% of under 2-year-olds used a mobile device.[13] Up until recently the American Academy of Pediatrics has recommended zero screen time for under 2-year-olds but they've decided to revise this in recognition that not all screen time is equal. It seems as though reading a child a story from an iPad is no different to reading from a book and interactive screen time is probably okay. American children these days average three hours a day in front of TV but five to seven hours of screen time including other devices.[14] But television in particular causes obesity because it induces both sedentary behavior *and* excess food consumption. Many studies confirm a positive relationship between hours of television watching and the prevalence of obesity in children. But is the rise in obesity due to less physical activity or more eating? The National Health and Nutrition Examination Survey in the United States asked 4,000 children between 8 and 16 years of age about diet and hours of television viewing. They found that as hours of television increased (10% of 11–13 year olds between 1988 and 1994 watched more than five hours of television a day), calorie intake also increased.[15]

A similar study using data from the New Zealand National Nutrition Survey from 2002 showed children and adolescents who watched more than two hours of television a day were twice as likely to drink soft drinks five times a week or more, and to eat hamburgers and fries at least once a week. Over the same period, 30% of the ads on television were for sweet snacks, 20% for drinks, and 15% for fast food restaurants.[16] In other words, the food that people eat more of when they are watching television is the food that is advertised on television.

For adolescents in particular, hours spent in front of the television are often at the expense of sleep. Experiments show that sleep deprivation is associated with increased levels of the hypothalamic hormone leptin as well as the hunger-inducing hormone ghrelin; subjects restricted to less than seven hours of sleep a night show corresponding rises in hunger and appetite. Quite how Margaret Thatcher managed to avoid obesity with her very small requirement for sleep I don't know because sleep deprivation is associated not only with weight gain but also with impaired glucose tolerance and vascular disease. Interestingly, the relationship between hours of sleep and weight is a U-shaped curve with both short and long hours of sleep associated with increased BMI—almost certainly the result of different mechanisms.[17] Obesity itself causes sleep disturbance too—most obviously obstructive sleep apnea.

New foods

Over a short period of time WHO has had to shift its attention from protein and calorie under-nutrition as a leading health concern to non-communicable diseases resulting from obesity. There are two aspects of dietary change involved in this change: a nutrition transition in developing countries, and the evolution in developed countries of the 'fast food nation'.[18]

In some developing countries we see the double burden of under-nutrition, usually affecting children, and over-nutrition or obesity affecting adults. This has been termed the nutrition transition paradox.[19] Two separate but related phenomena contribute to the nutrition transition in developing countries. The first is the increasing wealth of a nation and the second is globalization of diet. In the poorest countries significant proportions of the community are underweight and the wealthier people are normal weight. As wealth increases the better-off members of society start to become overweight or even obese. In time, though, the prevalence of obesity shifts to the poorer members of society—this is the pattern in the developed world currently. The globalization of diet leads to food becoming more energy dense. A big change has been the increased use of vegetable oils for cooking in countries like Africa and, worldwide, we are all eating sweeter food.[20] The final switch is from a carbohydrate or plant-based diet to one with a high proportion of animal protein. This last change is probably the best way to track nutrition transition across the globe. The average calorie intake in the developing world rose from 1,950 to 2,680 kilocalories per person per day between the early 1960s and 2005. Protein intake almost doubled going from 40 to 70 grams per day. Increasing the proportion of animal protein in the diet improves health for those who are chronically undernourished but the effect plateaus once the requirements for micronutrients such as iron and vitamins are met. After that more milk and meat in the diet leads to increasing amounts of cholesterol and saturated fat in the diet. An estimate based on data from the Food and Agriculture Organization of the United Nations (FAO) has the number of countries with intakes of cholesterol exceeding WHO recommendations increasing from 26 in 1961–63 to 64 in 1999–2001. The figures for total fat and saturated fat match these.[21] Even if you don't believe in the dangers of saturated fat (I do), this clearly represents an increase in energy density of the diet. Fat has 9 calories per gram while carbohydrate (and protein) has 4.

One way or another, diets worldwide have shifted from an emphasis on fruits and vegetables to animal protein and cereals, or seeds. Efficiencies in the production of protein (the agri-economy) are responsible for animal protein becoming cheaper but the emergence of the processed food industry has resulted in our eating things which are no longer identifiable as foods. The American space program may have kicked off our fascination with processed food with a stream of newspaper articles describing developments in astronauts' food throughout the 1960s. In 1962 we learned that Colonel John Glenn Junior on *Friendship 7* had a space snack that consisted of a beef-vegetable course followed by an applesauce course—both resembling toothpaste in tubes. It was described as being a bit like baby food but with adult sugar and seasonings added. By 1965 on *Gemini 4* the process of freeze-drying had become the standard method of preparing space food with water added to the plastic bag and the reconstituted food sucked through a straw. Other food seems to have been squashed into bite-sized lumps (bacon and egg, cubes of cheese) which were okay so long as they were transferred directly into the mouth from the bag. We learned that food in weightless conditions exploded into crumbs when exposed to the atmosphere—as happened on the first mission when someone smuggled a corned beef sandwich on board.

Food has of course been processed for thousands of years. Cooking makes food more digestible and converting olives to oil, grapes to wine, and adding natural yeasts to flour to produce leavening are other ancient forms of food processing. Freezing, drying, canning, salting, and so forth are ways in which food is minimally processed in order to make produce that grows in one season available in another (entirely redundant now with food being flown around the globe from wherever it's in season). Now we take animal protein, mince it up to produce a slurry, add starches, oils, salt, and other ingredients and then shape the substance in a mold so that it looks for all the world like a naturally occurring piece of meat. Chicken nuggets are the archetype and fish trimmings are transformed to crab-claw-imitating surimi, horse meat becomes beef patties, and milk is transformed to plastic-like sheets of pale yellow material called cheese. Snack foods and breakfast cereals take this one step further with food production that many are now calling 'ultra-processing.' Professor Carlos Monteiro from São Paulo categorizes food into three groups. In the type one category he puts natural foods or those which are minimally processed. Type two are ingredients such as nutrient-depleted oils, fats, sugar and sweeteners, flours, starch, and salt. Type three foods are products made up of type two ingredients. High-fructose corn syrup is an example of a type two food. This by-product of corn processing isn't something humans would have encountered without the benefit of a manufacturing process which essentially pre-digests corn. Corn syrup is more stable than other sugars and is now a major part of the modern diet. Type three foods are:

durable, accessible, convenient, attractive, ready-to-eat or ready-to heat products. These ultra-processed foods are formulated to reduce microbial deterioration (long shelf life), to be transportable for long distances, to be extremely palatable (high organoleptic quality) and often to be habit forming. Typically they are designed to be eaten anywhere—in fast-food establishments, at home instead of domestically prepared and cooked food, while watching television, at a desk or elsewhere at work, on the street, and while driving.[22]

None of this would probably matter, and you could probably argue for greater efficiency in the use of expensive animal protein, if it wasn't for the fact that the incorporation of flavoring agents and additives that enhance successful storage of these products makes them vastly less healthy than the original foods from which they were derived. Over and above that, the increased energy density means that these foods displace other healthy foods from the diet, resulting in a double whammy effect that reduces micronutrients in the diet.

Vegetables contain high levels of the healthy fatty acid omega 3, which is attractive to pests. Refining grains by removing the husks reduces spoiling but shifts the balance in the grain towards the unhealthy omega 6 fatty acids, which promote atherosclerosis or the build-up of plaque on arteries. It also increases the glycemic index of food by removing fiber. The glycemic index (GI) refers to the speed with which carbohydrates are broken down to simple sugars and absorbed. Once absorbed, insulin is required to shift the sugar into muscle and fat. If you have diabetes and faulty insulin production you learn to avoid high GI foods as your blood sugar shoots up within a short time of eating and a faulty pancreas can't cope. If instead you eat slow release or low GI foods, the conversion to sugar happens very slowly and even a failing pancreas might be able to release enough insulin to deal with what you've eaten.

Perhaps in recognition of the shortcomings of processed foods, manufacturers have started adding back the very things that processing took out. A cynic might say that consumers have become aware of these shortcomings and manufacturers have taken advantage of a marketing opportunity. Proclamations that foods such as marshmallows are cholesterol free, for example, suggests manufacturers are more interested in tapping into consumer concerns than actually producing healthier food. It is now routine to see these artificial foods with vitamins and an array of trace elements added—folate, vitamins C, D and A, iron and even fiber. But this doesn't turn these products back into food.

Marion Nestle, New York University Professor of Nutrition and public health advocate, and others describe this practice as a preoccupation with nutrients as opposed to food and this leads to a great deal of confusion as to what is healthy or not. Is an unadorned piece of fruit likely to be as good for you as a beautifully packaged carton of juice with extra vitamin C, and the ingredients and the percentage of daily requirements listed on the side? The problem is a lack of knowledge about what it is exactly that makes a fruit-and-vegetable-based diet healthier than one that is scarce in these items. It's suggested that the benefits come from anti-oxidants, vitamins, and so forth but it's likely that the whole is greater than the sum of its parts. A piece of fruit contains cellulose and pectin which may not directly contribute to nutrition but are important in slowing digestion and stomach emptying, so sugar is released relatively slowly into the bloodstream. Fruit juice on the other hand—even when freshly squeezed prior to drinking—is more like a sugar-sweetened cordial than a piece of fruit. The stuff in the carton therefore just hasn't got that essential fruitiness no matter how many 'nutrients' are added.

The very notion of processed food is based on the fallacy that you can deconstruct food then recreate it again in an improved form through modern technological processes. Some food additives are beneficial—for example, iodine in salt. Iodine deficiency is common throughout the world and leads to goiter and, in severe cases, to cretinism. Trace amounts of iodine are required to prevent these diseases and while public health measures can work, such as the adding of iodine to public wells in China to prevent cretinism in iodine-deficient regions, the most effective way of dealing with the deficiency is to add potassium iodide to salt. This practice began after the First World War and once the dose was right (initially it was too low), it has been remarkably effective. Similarly, vitamin D is added to milk to treat rickets in regions of high latitude (we make vitamin D in response to sunlight exposure) and folate to flour to prevent spina bifida. In these cases the food is used as a vector to distribute trace elements that are missing in the environment and, although some food purists object, most would see this as a public good that improves the health of the population.

The supermarket revolution

To a large degree supermarket chains are responsible for the development of a global diet. In New Zealand the first 'groceteria' opened in Dunedin in 1927. By 1958 'self-service' grocers made up 25% of the grocery stores in the country. The amount spent in New Zealand supermarkets has been stable at around NZ$4 billion a quarter since 2011,[23] which is close to the NZ$30 million *daily* the now defunct current affairs *Campbell Live* reported on 15 February 2013. In the United States, Walmart is the current exemplar of corporate business with 1.4 million employees in 2005 and estimated sales of a trillion dollars a year in 2013. Twenty million shoppers visit the store each day and it's the single largest US importer of Chinese goods. It's said that if Walmart was a country it would be China's eighth largest trading partner—ahead of Russia and Great Britain.[24] With operating budgets that exceed the gross domestic product of many countries, supermarkets have an enormous ability to influence the food chain for good or for bad. For example, in Brazil the supermarkets were responsible for increasing the sales of ultra-heat-treated dairy products so that the population had access to safe and inexpensive milk.

Corporations like Walmart, and Tesco in the United Kingdom, influence the earnings of a large proportion of the labor market by controlling the wages, not only of direct employees but also of those involved in the manufacturing and transportation of the goods sold. It used to be that the supplier or grower produced goods according to demand and growing conditions and the role of the retailer was simply to on-sell them. With the buying power of the large supermarket chains it's the retailer who now calls the shots. Growers' contracts can require the supply of vegetables grown at a loss. Access to supermarket shelving space means that the price of goods is set by the seller rather than the producer and we the consumers have our food-buying behavior manipulated in myriad ways, with price being the most obvious.

Supermarkets have a significant influence on our diet given they supply most of the food we eat. In 2005, 70% of the food bought by New Zealanders came from a supermarket—from one of the two chains which operate in the restricted market of a duopoly. Supermarkets' own brands, which used to be a cheaper version of normal product lines, now occupy a bigger share of the market—especially with regard to preprepared meals. I remember frozen TV dinners in the 1950s and 1960s; roast chicken and gravy in little compartments in aluminium foil trays—so exotic, and far too expensive for us to ever have at home. But a recent estimate of the average time taken to prepare a meal eaten at home is 15 minutes so something else is replacing home cooking. My 92-year-old father adds frozen vegetables to precooked meals but even families rely on pasta sauces, cooked chickens, salad mixes, and frozen pizzas to speed up dinner.

Supermarkets are also the source of most of the high-fat, high-sugar food and drink, with shelves of cheap snack foods, sweetened drinks and confectionery that are sold with a small profit margin but in vast quantities. An appreciation of the corporate heft of supermarkets has spawned a resistance movement. The Tescopoly Alliance cites the negative impacts of supermarket chains on farmers, workers worldwide, garment workers, UK workers, homeworkers, the environment, food poverty, healthiness of food, and animal welfare. The environmental issues include the cost of transporting food from the site of production (the other side of the world in some cases), the cost of transport for the shopper (1 in 10 car journeys in the United Kingdom are to buy food), the use of plastic bags and other packaging, and the effect of more than 300,000 tons of food waste each year.[25]

What environmental change matters most?

The life of a child growing up in Te Awamutu now (current population 12,000) compared to that of 40 or 50 years ago is different in more ways than we can describe. The transformation of ordinary existence for a child growing up in China or India over the same time period is even more dramatic. In determining which aspect correlates best with the sharp rise in obesity over the last 30 years, the evidence favors an increase in energy supply rather than a decrease in energy expenditure. Technological advances (combine harvesters, computers, electric vacuum cleaners, automatic washing machines, and leaf blowers, for example) have had the greatest impact on work-related and domestic energy expenditure over the last century. But history doesn't support the idea that mechanization is the major driver of the obesity epidemic. At the beginning of the nineteenth century the industrial revolution led to a dramatic rise in food production which was later enhanced by fertilizers and pesticides. In the first half of the twentieth century there was a measured reduction in food eaten as a result of further technological advances reducing energy requirements in the workplace and at home. This was especially obvious in the years immediately following the Second World War when there were weight and height gains in the population but reduced energy consumption. The matching of supply and demand ended in the 1960s and 1970s when the supply of food, stimulated by subsidies, started to outstrip demand.

The last 40 years have seen the commodification of food led by the fast food industry and supermarket giants in the context of free market ideology. These macro-economic drivers are discussed in more detail in the following chapter. The end result, however, has been an increase in the numbers of calories available in the food supply. In the United States, 3,200 calories per day per capita were available in 1980 which had risen to 3,900 by the year 2000.[26] While there have been an incredible number of changes to our environment over the course of my lifetime (60 years), it is eating more than we need to that has made us fat.

6

How the economics of food puts more of it on our plates

For baby boomers like me the world revolves around individuals. We value independence, self-reliance, and freedom of choice. We believe in a free market in which the supply of goods is dictated by the strength of our demand. Globalization means we buy food from everywhere in the world and, providing we can afford it, our diet is what we choose it to be. Or is it? The free market is supposed to empower the consumer but we hand this power over to multinational companies who in turn *create* demand (having worked out what sells). Yes, we get to choose this brand of chips over another, but larger forces determine the cheapness of chips and influence our preference for these over rice or taro. For individuals, personal factors, including wealth, contribute to the difference between one person's diet and the next, but farming and trade policies and macro-economic forces outside individual control determine what we eat as a population. If we want to overcome the obesity epidemic we need to regain control of the food systems not just the food.

Food rationing (eat less)

Prior to the Second World War, Britain imported 70% of its food, with New Zealand providing a sixth of its meat, a quarter of its butter, and half of its cheese. The population was vulnerable to starvation if supply lines were interrupted, as they were during the world wars, and funding the war effort meant less could be spent on the importation of food. Food shortages during the First World War had led to huge queues and outrageously inflated prices, so second time around the British government was better prepared, with ration booklets already printed in 1938. War was declared on 3 September 1939 and the Ministry of Food was reconstituted on 4 September. Campaigners like Sir John Boyd Orr were already working with the Ministry of Food, petitioning the government to improve the nutrition of the poor which had deteriorated as a result of the industrial revolution and urbanization. The defeat in the two Boer wars was blamed on the puny, undernourished fighting stock that made up the British Army of the time, so politicians were open to the idea of improving nutrition and rationing scarce supplies was one way of doing this. Everyone had to produce a food coupon before they were able to buy bacon, ham, fats, cheese, sugar, and sugar products, and milk and eggs were 'quasi-rationed.' Although supplies were less than ideal (fueling a vigorous black market), it did mean this food was available to the poor, which wouldn't have been the case if market forces controlled supply. In 1940 Frederick Marquis, Baron

Woolton, was appointed as Minister of Food. A former social worker and managing director of the Lewis chain of department stores, he had no prior experience in politics or government but was used to communicating with customers and he set about educating the population about nutrition. Famous for Woolton pie (wholemeal crust, vegetable filling), he led a comprehensive program promoting fruit and vegetables. There were posters and songs featuring Dr Carrot 'the Children's best friend' and Potato Pete 'I make good soup,' and parks all over the country became allotments for growing vegetables. The Dig for Victory campaign was waged throughout the war with poster displays, recipes, and even anthems. People set up pig clubs, pooling vegetables to feed an animal for slaughter in someone's back garden, and anyone who could kept chickens. From a purely health point of view, Britain's diet was never better.[1]

Meat was rationed in Britain for 14 years, until 1954, and over this time the supply of food varied from year to year. Between 1943 and 1949 the Ministry of Food monitored the calorie intake and body weights of the working-class population to see if the food supply was adequate. Each year they visited the homes of 20,000–30,000 people, inspecting their larders and asking about food purchases to calculate the calorie content of their diet. In those days there was no need to consider food eaten outside of the home and they made the decision to ignore food provided for visitors. They also weighed the household members and clearly documented that between 1940 and 1943 and again between 1946 and 1947 a diet containing less than 2,900 calories a day resulted in weight loss. During 1944 the average calorie intake was 3,000 and there was a sharp rise in weights. An average intake of 2,900 calories kept the weight of the population stable.[2] What makes this data interesting is not the fact that people lose weight when food is short but that they become overweight in the face of an excess. In other words, you can manipulate the average weight of the population by adjusting the food supply.

In the United States food rationing began in 1942 and ended in 1946. M. F. K. (Mary Francis Kennedy) Fisher was a witty, sophisticated food writer who spent the early years of her marriage in France. Back in the US in 1942, she wrote *How to Cook a Wolf*, an exhortation to eat well despite lean times, and chapters included 'How to Catch a Wolf,' 'How to be Cheerful Though Starving,' and 'How to Pray for Peace'. In the foreword for a later edition of the book she wrote:

> There are very few men and women, I suspect, who cooked and marketed their way through the past war without losing forever some of the nonchalant extravagance of the twenties. They will feel, until their final days on earth, a kind of culinary caution: butter, no matter how unlimited, is a precious substance not lightly to be wasted; meats too, and eggs, and all the far-brought spices of the world, take on a new significance, having once been so rare.[3]

How times have changed.

But, despite the efforts of Fisher and others, when the US government conducted a household survey of food consumption in the 1960s they found that Americans weren't eating well—that the diet was deficient in many nutrients. Not only that, but many people on low incomes were hungry.

Production-led agricultural policy (eat more)

This finding led to the Department of Agriculture implementing policy changes to get people eating more meat, milk, and eggs. Marion Nestle in her book *Food Politics* describes this era as one in which the population was encouraged to 'eat more.'[4] Aided by federal support, American farmers were encouraged to not only fatten up America but to feed the world. What they were told to grow was corn, wheat, and soy beans. These foods lend themselves to large-scale production, easy storage, and long-distance shipping. Research was directed to improving efficiency and harvest yields, which in the case of corn saw a 600% increase in the bushels per acre between the 1920s and the 1990s.[5] As production rose, the price, of course, dropped. Less efficient small farms were amalgamated into enormous ventures growing a single product, rather like today's New Zealand dairy farms. Most importantly, these changes mark the start of an era when food was grown not in response to demand, but as a commodity for which a need would have to be created.

Food subsidies (keep eating)

The idea of the free market is that supply adjusts to match demand. In 1950s New Zealand the export economy was based on sheep farming with good prices being paid for wool and sheep meat. When Britain entered the European Economic Community in 1973, New Zealand lost its export market overnight. While new markets were being sought the government-subsidized farmers, providing up to 40% of their income by the early 1980s. In 1984, though, the government removed all subsidies leaving farmers to compete with the still heavily subsidized agriculture sectors in Europe and the US. This led to great gains in efficiency, particularly in the dairy industry, and 95% of the milk produced today is exported with most of it going to China. The change in markets has seen vast acreages converted from sheep to dairy farming.

But many countries haven't taken such a staunch free market approach and subsidies to farmers persist as a result of powerful lobbying by the farming sector. One example is the 1996 Farm Act passed by the US federal government to provide subsidies to farmers struggling to survive in the face of falling crop prices. In order to limit the number of farmers receiving funding, the payments were based on both the historical *usage* of the land (for eligible crops) and historical commodity prices. These restrictions compounded the problem further because, in order to be eligible for the program, farmers had to keep growing the same crops and were specifically prohibited from growing wild rice, fruit, nuts, and all vegetables other than lentils, mung beans, and dry peas. Not only did this prevent diversification but it guaranteed continued production of food in excess of demand, which resulted in further drops in prices and the need for increased subsidies. It's hardly surprising that the United States overproduces cheap calories in the form of grains and sugars while underproducing fruit and vegetables. While some of the excess production is exported, the distorted agricultural output has its maximum effect on the domestic food supply and in turn on the diet of the local population.

Careful tracking of the spending on food subsidies by Mike Russo and Dan Smith from the US Public Interest Research Group led them to the following conclusions: since 1995

American taxpayers have paid $292.5 billion in agricultural subsidies. Most of this goes to large, already profitable players, with $178.5 billion going to just 3.8% of farmers. Of this, $19.2 billion went to subsidize the production of corn sweeteners, corn starch, and soy oils. These nutritionally barren products are compared to apples for which the taxpayer has paid a mere $689 million to promote over the same period. In the United States, apples are the only fruit or vegetable to receive significant support for production.[6] In 2002 the US Department of Agriculture estimated that between 1985 and 2002 the average person had increased their intake by 300 calories. Of these extra calories 24% were from fat, 23% from added sugars, and 46% from (mostly refined) grains.[7]

The United States isn't the only country to pay subsidies to farmers; the European Union spends €2 billion a year maintaining milk production at 20% beyond demand at twice the market value.[8] Incentives for export and local consumption are now required to deal with the oversupply. Excess milk in Sweden ends up in the school milk program and because full-fat is more heavily subsidized than low-fat, children are given the less healthy, high-fat version. In this way the subsidy contributes both to the energy density of children's diets and to heart disease as a result of the saturated fat.[9]

Some countries subsidize food prices for the *consumer* as a way to alleviate poverty, using this as a mechanism, like taxation, for influencing consumption without necessarily altering production costs. While these subsidies too are controversial (in terms of efficacy) they don't have the same potential to pervert the agricultural economy in the long term as production subsidies do. Food is cheaper now than it has ever been before and more abundant, with evidence that food supplies overall will be sufficient for the next 25 years at least. The FAO predicts that in 2050 the percentage of the population living in countries with an average food consumption of more than 3,000 calories per day will rise from 28% currently to 52%. Those living in countries where the average is under 2,500 calories per day will fall from 35% to 2.6%.[10] The incentives have shifted from increasing production to increasing consumption as a way of maintaining demand and therefore market prices. Waste is also increasing but, by and large, our response to excess food is that we eat it.

Creating demand

Corn production deserves special mention because it provides the best example of a food grown in quantities far greater than the global demand and of the inventive approaches taken to subsequently dispose of it. When corn was first grown by settlers in the midwestern US states at the beginning of the twentieth century, its prime role was as food. A poster from 1918 exhorts housewives to 'Serve Some Way Every Meal.' Today only 1% is eaten as recognizable corn, up to 12% ends up in food such as corn chips or in the form of high-fructose corn syrup, and 70% is consumed as feed for livestock raised for slaughter, poultry, and fish. According to the National Corn Growers Association 2013 report, 'many household products contain corn, including paints, candles, fireworks, drywall, sandpaper, dyes, crayons, shoe polish, antibiotics, and adhesives.'[11] This list provides just a hint of corn's versatility. To read Michael Pollan's *Omnivore's Dilemma* is to be truly scared by the pervasiveness of this plant in our modern lives. According to Pollan more than 10,000 food items in the supermarket contain corn and in addition pesticides, waxes, and materials from which the supermarket is built are also often corn-derived.[12]

One way of using up the corn biomass is to ferment it into ethanol and to use this as an additive to gasoline. But ethanol is a much less efficient source of energy and when production and transport costs are taken into account, unadulterated gasoline is cheaper. If properly calculated, the energy required for the growing, harvesting, manufacturing, and transport costs of ethanol production from corn results in a negative energy balance. If the environmental costs of using fossil fuels for this purpose are added in, the cost is even higher.[13]

Putting aside the issue of corn production displacing fruit and other vegetable production, the main concern from a dietary point of view is the conversion of the carbohydrate to corn syrup. This is an extremely stable compound with a long shelf life and it's cheaper than sugar derived from cane or beets. For these reasons corn syrup has made its way into the array of processed foods that Americans eat every day. In addition a typical 12 fluid ounce bottle of soft drink contains 16 teaspoons of sugar derived from corn syrup. This is a problem in terms of quantity alone, with the American Heart Association recommending no more than six teaspoons of added sugar a day for women and nine for men.

Milk may be the new corn when it comes to commoditized food. New Zealand is almost entirely dependent on the dairy sector for export earnings, and while farming is not subsidized the industry receives strong political support. Fonterra, a New Zealand dairy co-operative, collects 22 billion liters of milk a year and much of this is made into milk powder. Like corn syrup, it has a long shelf life and lends itself to processed food production.

But the exemplar of creating a market for milk is the huge multinational company Nestlé. Starting out as a producer of condensed milk and infant formula, it now manufactures ice cream, confectionery, snack food, pet food, and drinks with annual sales of around US$30 billion. The most controversial aspect of dairy food marketing is the promotion of infant formula in emerging markets. Countries like China and Indonesia have low and falling breastfeeding rates as a result of aggressive targeting of pregnant women with sophisticated campaigns, free samples, and gifts. Healthcare workers are easily bribed for details of expectant mothers, and while China banned the provision of free formula samples in birthing units in reality this continues to be the norm. This behavior prompted the formation of the International Baby Food Action Network and the misdemeanors of manufacturers of infant formula are described in their publication 'Breaking the Rules.' The Danis Tanović movie *Tigers* is based on the story of Syed Aamir Raza, a former salesman for Nestlé who blew the whistle on his employer after he failed to negotiate changes in the way the company marketed infant formula in Pakistan.

The market for infant formula has been threatened by the deaths in China from melamine contamination as well as by the efforts of governments to promote breastfeeding. This has pushed milk powder companies to create a totally new range of products in order to maintain sales (and profits). These products, called 'growing up milks' (GUMs), are milk drinks with additives and are designed for toddlers. Another range of products has been created for pregnant women, or breastfeeding mothers. Supply in response to demand? I don't think so.

Free trade agreements – free for whom?

In theory, the liberalization of food trade between countries benefits everyone by increasing economic growth and reducing food prices. In reality, the outcome is often different.[14] Some blame insufficient liberalization for the failure of free trade agreements to deliver economic prosperity (powerful countries holding onto subsidies) while others argue that the very nature of the agreements favors richer countries. For example, in order to join the North American Free Trade Agreement (NAFTA), Mexico had to cease subsidies on its corn production, while the United States could retain theirs. In the 10 years since this agreement was put in place, 1.3 million Mexican farmers have gone bankrupt and Mexico has gone from self-sufficient corn production to now importing half of what it needs. Paradoxically it was the cheap price of corn from the US which put small farmers out of business but prices have now risen in response to reduced local supply and in 2008 prices tripled, contributing further to poverty.[15]

In addition to the effect on local agriculture, NAFTA opened the floodgates for the exportation of junk foods and soft drinks from the United States. Mexico now has obesity rates exceeding that of the US at 35% of the adult population, and this is matched by rapidly increasing soft drink sales. The average per capita consumption of Coca-Cola in 2010 was about 42 gallons per person in comparison with about 26 gallons per person in the US. Expansion of export markets has undoubtedly contributed to the globalization of diet, and for many of the smaller or weaker FTA member countries this is associated with the loss of food sovereignty, and the struggle to retain traditional agricultural practices and diet, particularly for indigenous populations (see page 106).

Pacific Island countries provide insight into the complexities of dealing with more powerful trading partners. Most small nations in the South Pacific aren't yet members of free trade organizations but they have complex relationships with countries like Australia, New Zealand, and the United States, who provide aid as well as being trading partners. New Zealand, for example, makes a significant contribution to the financial stability of Samoa by purchasing up to 50% of the country's exports (mostly coconut products) as well as supplying 35–40% of Samoa's imports. In 2007 the New Zealand Labour government rejected recommendations to ban the export of mutton flaps (which in New Zealand would be made into pet food) and other fatty meats, citing free trade commitments. At a Pacific Parliamentary and Politics Forum in Wellington in 2013, members of the Samoan Parliament again appealed to the New Zealand government to stop the export of mutton flaps, which were described as wreaking havoc on health.[16] The pleas are falling on deaf ears it would seem and Samoa is losing the battle on other fronts as well. Turkey tails, exported from the US, are 35% fat and are cheap compared to locally caught fish and fresh vegetables. In 2011 the Prime Minister Tuilaepa Sailele Malielegaoi was quoted as saying, 'The turkey should bring its own tail to Samoa. It's no good somebody else chowing the turkey and then sending the tail to Samoa.'[17] Sadly, in response to their bid to join the World Trade Organization (WTO), Samoa was advised that targeting individual products contravened the rules and they were given 12 months to remove the turkey tail ban. Individuals are now able to import these for personal use—with or without turkey attached.

Mutton flaps are up to 50% fat. Fiji banned their importation on health grounds before the WTO was formed and, on becoming a member of the organization, New Zealand threatened to refer Fiji to the dispute settlement body for contravening the policy of free trade. In Tonga, people eat New Zealand mutton flaps 2.3 times a week on average. They are significantly cheaper than local or traditional sources of protein. The Tongan prime minister 'Ulukalala Lavaka Ata said they were 'hardly edible by the health standards of New Zealand,' but Tonga is an observer to the WTO and if they want acceptance as a full member the mutton flaps can't be banned according to the rules of the GATT (General Agreement on Tariffs and Trade).[18]

In November 2015 governments of 12 countries including New Zealand and the US agreed on the text for the Trans-Pacific Partnership Agreement (TPPA). This agreement has attracted huge opposition, with worldwide protests from groups with concerns ranging from increased costs of medicines to extensions of copyright. The international climate group 350.org. fears that legislation designed to curb pollution and reduce greenhouse gas emissions will be subject to attack as the terms of the agreement allow corporations to sue governments for loss of profits. Similarly, anyone can see that the introduction of legislation such as soft drink or fat taxes, zoning restrictions on fast food outlets, or restrictions on advertising might all (hopefully) result in a reduction of sales of these products and therefore profit. If the affected companies are huge fast food or soft drink multinationals, New Zealand—like Samoa and Fiji— might find that it is unable to enact public health legislation without facing huge financial penalties. Even the US, the big player in the game, might lose out against the multinationals, and farmers in particular are watching the developments with considerable unease.

The TPPA agreement was signed in Auckland on 4 February 2016 amid much protest—just as this book was going to press. To come into effect, it now requires ratification by all countries, including passing through the US Congress.

Emerging junk food markets

There are signs that in many parts of the developed world obesity rates are starting to level off—particularly for children. The children of today are growing up in a world already saturated with high-energy processed food and drink. For example, I'm writing this while sitting on a plane flying from San Francisco to Boston. Food on the flight is available in the form of snack boxes. This is what is in the 'classic' snack box:

- Mott's applesauce
- Pepperidge Farm goldfish crackers
- pepperoni
- gourmet cheddar cheese spread
- more crackers
- candy
- Oreo cookies.

There are free soft drinks to go with the snack boxes.

Many people now eat these pseudo-foods as their usual sources of sustenance. In less developed and poorer countries this isn't yet the case; traditional food is still being eaten, but not for long. A posting from William Reed Business Media refers to the business plans of several cookie and confectionery producers who are targeting the fast-growing markets of India, China, Africa, and the Middle East. Irene Rosefeld, the CEO of the mega cookie, chip, and chocolate company Mondelēz, is quoted as saying 'as GDP per capita grows it drives consumption of chocolates, biscuits and other snacks; that's a great recipe for sustainably high growth rate.'[19] So confident are they of double-digit growth in these markets they are investing US$600 million to promote these products in the developing world. When I get to Boston I'll be in an enlightened city where the sale of sweetened drinks is banned in city-owned premises (the population spends far less than the national average on junk food per year).

Similarly, cigarette smoking is prohibited in restaurants and bars and most public venues across the US, but cigarette companies are pouring money into the developing world, targeting children and women in particular, as a means of maintaining sales. At the same time Mondelēz, Hershey's, Nestlé, and Kraft are working to ensure that Indians are chewing gum, the Chinese are eating chocolate, and the whole world is eating Oreo cookies.

Emerging markets increase the demand not only for junk food and confectionery but for meat and grain as well. As these societies move away from traditional diets to a Western one, it is predicted that the worldwide production of meat will need to increase by 85% between 2000 and 2030. Rearing livestock puts huge pressure on the environment (estimated to contribute 20% of global warming), and beef is the most expensive form of dietary protein. Although food on a global level is still plentiful and relatively inexpensive, there is a clear separation between the cost of healthy and unhealthy food. UK food prices between 2002 and 2008 have generally increased at a faster rate than the consumer price index (CPI), with the ranking from greatest to least price rise being: bread, fresh milk, vegetables, beef, then cookies and cakes. Soft drinks have risen at a rate *lower* than the CPI.[20] This data alone provides an explanation for the deterioration in the quality of diet in Britain at least.

The fight to retain food sovereignty

La Via Campesina, the way of the peasant, is a militant movement formed 20 years ago with the aim of supporting small local food producers and resisting colonization by global food giants. Their aim is to ensure the rights to use and manage lands, water, seeds, livestock, and biodiversity are in the hands of food producers not the corporate sector. They see their enemies as being not only multinational companies but also the World Bank, the International Monetary Fund, and the WTO.[21]

With this in mind, we need to watch what happens to quinoa. This highly nutritious grain is the staple of the Andean region of South America and grows well in areas of low moisture. The UN recognized 2012 as 'the year of quinoa,' and the worldwide interest in this grain has the potential to significantly improve the economies of both Peru and Bolivia, where most of the world's supplies are grown. The success of quinoa is being celebrated as an example of treasuring local cuisine over global food and also of the general excellence of Peru's produce and food culture. At the moment quinoa is highly fashionable (you can buy it in upmarket food stores in Manhattan and Auckland) and expensive, but farmers around the world from Africa to Europe are starting to grow it so this may change quite quickly. It doesn't take much imagination to envisage the development of a scenario similar to that of corn production in Mexico. If modern agricultural techniques allow quinoa to be grown cheaply in other parts of the world, and free trade agreements allow unrestricted access to the Peruvian market, the domestic population could well face bankruptcies and subsequent price rises.

Optimists are comparing Peruvians to the French in their respect for local food. France has relatively low rates of obesity, perhaps as a result of strategies introduced a couple of decades ago when the highest density of McDonald's restaurants was to be found in Paris. These strategies included a rigorous healthy school lunch program. Children are not encouraged to bring their own food to school and vending machines in schools are banned. Soft drinks are taxed and there is a new proposal to ban free refills of soft drinks in fast food outlets. Meanwhile, back in Bolivia the small farmers are getting good money for their grain—which they are spending on beer and fast food. For the local populace, quinoa is already becoming too expensive for those on low incomes. They are making do with the cheap processed food that the rest of the world eats. In order to avoid the pitfalls faced by Mexico, local governments in Peru and Bolivia might need to bolster their endorsement of quinoa producers through regulation of the global food market—such as occurs in France.

What's gone wrong with food policy?

Postwar agricultural policies and free trade agreements from the 1980s onward are in part a response to the privation experienced in many countries during the Second World War. While the early driver to produce more food might have been to improve population health, agricultural policies are increasingly contributing to non-communicable diseases. On the one hand, WHO and governmental health departments throughout the world are imploring individuals to eat more fruit and vegetables and to consume less of the nutrient-poor, calorie-dense foods that contribute to obesity. At the same time agriculture and trade policies have the reverse effect. Despite decades of evidence that the greatest influence on the diet of the population is the quantity and nature of the food available on a macro-economic level, we are surprised when individuals eat badly in an environment where bad food is plentiful and cheap. Finally, we are reluctant to interfere with the free market and protect the individual by limiting the sale of junk food, but happy to step in and contribute to the *production* of junk food when the same free market fails the farmer.

So the scene has been set for food producers to exploit the market in pursuit of profits. Fast food chains were among the first to take advantage of this environment and the skills they developed and the success they achieved are described in the next chapter.

7

How we're sold on junk food

Eric Schlosser's classic book *Fast Food Nation* describes the evolution of the fast food industry with a particular emphasis on McDonald's.[1] He writes about the innovation and initiative Ray Kroc brought to the company in 1955 but goes on to expose the seamier aspects of its success, and his book is largely seen as an attack on the fast food industry. We are still grappling with the role fast food plays in the rise of obesity and, more importantly, whether its producers are friend or foe when it comes to providing solutions. When I talk about 'the food industry' I'm not using the term accurately to include the growers and sellers of fresh produce. I'm referring to processed food and drink—the stuff Gareth Morgan and Geoff Simmons call fake food in their book *Appetite for Destruction*.[2] If our eating patterns match those of Europeans, about 70% of our calories now come from these highly industrially processed foods.[3]

Acknowledging that listed food companies are required by law to deliver a profit to shareholders might exonerate some of their inventive methods for expanding markets and creating demand, but perhaps it rules them out as true partners when the solution to obesity is for people to eat less of their products. Can we rely on the food industry to use their skills and resources to get the population eating small amounts of healthy food, or is this akin to asking the fox to behave well in the hen house? The consumer needs a good understanding of marketing techniques in order to determine whether members of the food industry are genuine when they say they want to help. Examining the response of industry to initiatives such as food labeling and watching what they are doing in the developing world will also help us to decide if they are trustworthy.

The science of marketing

An advertisement on the back of a bus shows crackers in the shape of a guitar. This highlights how the processed food industry has it all over fresh food producers. Not only do they start with really cheap ingredients and large advertising budgets but the very nature of processed food means products can be made in cute shapes and attractive colors, and they can also be fine-tuned to have the right amount of fat, salt, and sweet to trigger a predictable taste response. Not for them years of cross-breeding to get a sweeter apple or a crisper lettuce. New Zealand's voluntary health star ratings on processed foods, introduced in 2014, are based on nutrient profiling and already food technologists are calculating what reformulations will achieve the highest rating for the least effort. We've come a long way from the iced animal crackers of my childhood and as the science of food technology has advanced so too has the science of marketing.

Otago University Professor Janet Hoek is an expert on irony in the medieval poem *Beowulf* but she subsequently left behind literature to pass over to the dark side (her term) of the world of marketing. She leads research in marketing and public policy and spills the beans on industry techniques. The first point she makes is that the ubiquity of fast food ads and the frequency with which they appear is a problem in itself because this fosters the impression that foods high in salt, sugar, and fat are part of a 'normal' diet. Another point she makes is that food is different to other products where the amount that can be consumed is limited and the goal of advertising is to make us switch brands. It's difficult to make people use more shampoo or gas but by the use of things like date-limited discounts, free upsizing, two-for-one deals, and so forth you can persuade people to eat more food.[4]

Professor Philip James, advisor to WHO, is a nutrition expert who started his career dealing with child starvation but has spent the last four decades fighting obesity. In his lectures he describes the use of science and technology to maximize sales: things like eye-tracking spectacles worn by mock supermarket shoppers so the length of time lingering over a particular item can be recorded as a means of evaluating changes in product packaging, price, or placement on the shelves. This information, along with sales data, is used to optimize placement in the store. It's no coincidence that the first items we see when we walk into a supermarket are the high-profit goods; that basic pantry items like tea and coffee

111

share the aisle with treats like potato chips and confectionery; or that small packets of sweets and chocolates—ideal for impulse purchases—line the checkouts.

Then there's the fantastic *range* of advertising media. Television advertising is still the mainstay but online advertising now accounts for one advertising dollar in five and is growing fast. In addition to online shopping sites, many stores buy advertisement side-bars that are programmed to roughly align with our internet searching. Tesco (the world's third largest retailer) is going to have scanning cameras on their gas station forecourts to categorize shoppers by age and sex so that advertisements showing on screens inside are tailored to the individual.[5] There is print media (all those mailbox flyers) and radio but I've seen soft drinks advertised on the back of buses, on handles you hold onto in subway trains, on the risers of stairs, bus shelters, the roofs of private dwellings, hoardings around sports arenas, and banners towed through the sky behind planes. The problem would be bad enough if we just stopped there but this is the tame stuff—these are all examples of things that we recognize as advertisements, so what about the rest?

Food advertising linked to sports is the perfect strategy because you get strong brand association of a product with a universally approved of activity. This is called the halo effect. In New Zealand sponsorship is mostly restricted to televised sports and little goes to sports clubs,[6] the exception being the sponsorship of junior soccer by McDonald's. Coke NZ launched Get Up and Go, which purports to promote cycling to teenagers by giving away free bikes. Quite apart from the halo effect, sponsoring sports events is a great way to maximize your audience. That is why a 30-second Super Bowl advertisement costs $4 million.

Using sporting heroes to promote your product is even more powerful. Researchers in the US selected athletes using their high rankings on the Bloomberg Business Week's 2010 endorsement value and found 23.8% were promoting food and drinks. When analyzed further it was seen that 79% of the food products were for junk food and 93.4% of the beverages had 100% of the calories from added sugar. The target audience for TV ads with sports personalities promoting food or drink is adolescents.[7] In Britain David Beckham advertised Pepsi and Burger King, the cricketer Shane Warne promoted McDonald's in Australia, and for a brief time cyclist Sarah Ulmer was persuaded to describe McDonald's as healthy food on New Zealand television. Most egregious is the current pairing of New Zealand's most cherished All Blacks rugby team with Coke. Do these sports celebrities actually consume the products they promote? We're never told. Politicians are keen to promote sports as the solution to obesity and naively (or disingenuously) suggest food industry sponsorship as an example of a partnership to solve the problem. It was this alignment of so many vested interests that led to the coup of a McDonald's and Coca-Cola sponsored London Olympics in 2012. During the Ashes campaign in Australia the commercial partnership of Kentucky Fried Chicken and Cricket Australia resulted in heavy advertisement of the 'tower burger.' To work off the calories contained in this burger you'd have to play two to three hours of continuous cricket, while most supporters are watching from the couch.

Selling to children

It's generally accepted that directly advertising to children under the age of 12 is wrong because they don't understand the difference between factual information and advertorial intent; most countries have some sort of regulation (even if only industry self-regulation) that acknowledges this. Sweden, Norway, and Quebec in Canada prohibit advertising anything at all to children under the age of 12. Personally I find the notion that adults are unaffected by advertisements farcical but it's certainly the case that an 8-year-old will treat *Sesame Street* or an advertisement for McDonald's as equally informative. The real problem is that even when so-called age restrictions are in place, they are a joke. There may be no advertising associated with the children's programs shown up until 5 p.m. at night (on New Zealand television) but the peak time for children to watch television is much later. If you really want to protect children under the age of 12 you need to ban advertisements for junk food until 9 p.m. In the United States children between the ages of 6 and 11 see on average 12.7 food ads a day and 86% of these are for unhealthy food.[8]

Although it hasn't yet eventuated, the clamor to restrict junk food and soft drink advertising on television is increasing. But so too is marketing via the internet. It's here that fast food companies are able to target children of all ages through 'adver-gaming.' They advertise on kids' websites like Nick.com and CartoonNetwork.com and have mobile apps with cute fluffy cartoon characters and subtle brand iconography. During my daily commute on the Waiheke Island ferry I see small children playing games and watching cartoons on iPads and smartphones.

A study by internet software company AVG found that more (19%) preschool children are able to use smartphone apps than (11%) tie their own shoe laces. (At least they'll be able to watch a YouTube video to help with that.) The point of advergaming is that often the links with products are subliminal. Look up McDonald's on the net and you see cheerful cartoon jingles about eating fruit and dairy products. The likelihood of a child associating McDonald's with eating fresh fruit is remote—everyone knows that Happy Meals are about burgers and fries. In addition there are games, competitions, and apps where you can enter quizzes and receive rewards, as well as Facebook accounts and Twitter—Coca-Cola and McDonald's have millions of followers. To test the effect of these strategies a group of researchers provided free food to 7–10-year-olds playing advergames; they found the kids ate more when playing games that advertised food.[9]

The use of cartoon characters and toys in marketing is increasingly controversial though it's an old ploy. When I was a child the cornflakes packets had crude plastic toys buried in among the golden flakes and this made Weet-Bix—with their color cards—a very sad second best. Cereal manufacturers have been outstripped by McDonald's in particular with the toys in Happy Meals. If anyone doubts the efficacy of this as a sales tool, read the story about the Teenie Beany Baby toys in *Fast Food Nation*. Schlosser points out that Happy Meals are aimed at children between the ages of 3 and 9 and within a week of this hugely successful promotion, four Happy Meals were sold for every child in that age group in America. Many countries now ban toys unless the meals they accompany meet certain nutritional standards but in many more this has been successfully contested by McDonald's. In April 2015, in New Zealand, Burger

115

King announced it will remove toys from its children's meals but McDonald's says it has no plans to follow suit.

Perhaps the biggest problem, as suggested by Janet Hoek, is the sheer volume of advertising. A report funded by the Robert Wood Johnson Foundation and carried out by the Yale Rudd Center for Food Policy and Obesity provides the following information:

- On the internet McDonald's placed 34 million display ads for Happy Meals per month.
- Fast food restaurants placed 6 billion ads on Facebook in 2012.
- In 2012 US fast food restaurants spent $4.6 billion in total on all advertising, an 8% increase from 2009.
- McDonald's spends 2.7 times as much to advertise its products ($972 million) as all fruit, vegetable, bottled water, and milk advertisers combined.[10]

As if that wasn't enough, advertisers make you feel small. At least according to underground artist Banksy:

> People are taking the piss out of you every day. They butt into your life, take a cheap shot at you and then disappear. They leer at you from tall buildings and make you feel small. They make flippant comments from buses that imply you're not sexy enough and that all the fun is happening somewhere else. They are on TV making your girlfriend feel inadequate. They have access to the most sophisticated technology the world has ever seen and they bully you with it. They are The Advertisers and they are laughing at you . . .[11]

'Fat free and 100% natural': Why labels matter

Australia and New Zealand share a food code and in 2010 the two governments jointly commissioned a review of food labeling law and policy. Food was already labeled with compulsory back-of-pack nutrient information, but this is so hard for most people to understand that in one survey a third of shoppers weren't able to identify the main ingredient from the list.[12] When asked to consider *front-of-pack* labels, such as traffic lights, with good food labeled green and bad labeled red, the submissions from the health sector and the food industry were diametrically opposed.[13] Many food manufacturers had their own system, with nutrients described in terms of the percentage of daily requirements per serving. Whether this very complicated system was designed to fend off regulated labeling or to simply confuse the shopper I don't know. More importantly, the loosely regulated labeling by manufacturers allows them to make claims that serve as potent marketing tools.

Professor Sandra Jones from the University of Wollongong describes these in her blog post 'Fat free and 100% natural: seven food labeling tricks exposed.' She covers such claims as 'no added sugar' on a fruit smoothie which is still sugar-loaded with over five teaspoons per seven fluid ounces. And the ridiculous statement that 'candy snakes are cholesterol-free.' It also seems there is nothing to stop producers claiming something is good for you when it's not. She describes cookies sold at her local gym which are simply labeled 'healthy' but actually contain more fat, salt, and sugar than the others on sale. Chips are described as being *lower* in salt or fat or calories but compared to what? One manufacturer has a chip brand that is lower in fat than their

other chip brand but both are higher than most competitors.'
A brand of packaged cheese has a large label describing the
product as 100% natural with no added flavors or colors—but
this should be true of all cheese.[14] These claims sound suspiciously
like those from an earlier era of tobacco advertising: 'Lucky
Strike. It's toasted.'

In the United States, the FDA only requires calorie labeling to
be accurate to within 20% and any amount of fat or sugar under
0.5 grams is allowed to be listed as 0 grams. Products advertised as made with 'wholegrains' or 'real fruit' may have these as
minuscule additions. And it is highly unlikely that the FDA will
intervene even if the error is greater. Enforcing these regulations
isn't a priority.

So what does work? The short answer is an *interpretive* label
that tells you whether this is a good or bad thing for you to eat.
Because some shoppers are particularly interested in nutrients
such as fat, or sugar (if you have diabetes) or salt, most of these
types of labels include a traffic light rating of red, orange, or green
for the separate components. New Zealand and Australia's star
rating system is based on 'nutrient profiling,' where positive
marks are given for nutrients and negative for harmful components so that a food ends up with a single score.[15] The score
could also be used as the basis for a variable food tax or of determining restrictions on marketing. But its most likely effect will
be to encourage manufacturers to reformulate their products in
order to avoid a punitive rating. Most importantly, when buying
processed or 'invented' food made up of goodness knows what,
consumers deserve to know whether it's healthy or not.

The food manufacturers disagree. So violently, in fact, that
they are prepared to spend huge sums of money lobbying to block

interpretive labels. This was most visible in Europe where it was estimated by the spokesperson for the confederation of food and drink manufacturers, the CIAA, that they spent €1 billion promoting the alternative daily allowance label.[16] When this was exposed in the blog Brussels Sunshine there was all sorts of back-tracking, with the CIAA attempting to deny that it was a lobbying organization and later trying to downplay the amount of money spent. The CIAA has more than 21 full-time staff and 10 accred-ited lobbyists at the European Parliament with an annual wage bill of €1.8 million. Another industry group calling itself Alliance for Food Industry put leaflets on the desks of all members of the European Parliament urging them to vote against amendments to the food information proposal.[17] No surprise, then, that despite public health experts and health-related government officials pushing hard for a traffic light labeling system, the proposal was decisively rejected.

Buying science

In her book *Food Politics* Marion Nestle exposes the techniques used to ensure that government policy favors the food industry.[18] Trade organizations for the explicit purpose of lobbying poli-ticians on the behalf of their members have always existed, but these are being joined by front groups which act not as lobbyists but more as public relations campaigners. In addition, food pro-ducers rebranding themselves as 'nutrition companies' are hiding behind pseudo-scientific advisory boards. The Center for Food Safety, an environmental advocacy organization keeping tabs on the food industry, offers tips on how to spot an organization that is really a front group. Most important is the funding source but words like 'alliance' and 'council' in the title are a clue and so too are their strategies. Typically these front groups pretend that they are sticking up for the small guy, that they have grassroots support, and they make out the opposition are extremists by calling them 'food Nazis.' They scaremonger by saying that new policies will result in job losses or higher prices and they buy science by paying for research without disclosure of conflicts of interest.[19]

An example of buying science can be seen in a recent article in *PLoS One*, a peer-reviewed open access online journal. The authors analyzed the reported food intake from more than 60,000 participants in the US National Health and Nutrition Examination Survey and determined that the results were too unreliable to use in formulating public policy in relation to obesity. Who would have a vested interest in discounting this huge body of nutritional data you may wonder. It turns out that the analysis was paid for by Coca-Cola and two of the three authors received funding from Coca-Cola.[20] We have Marion Nestle to thank for continuing vigilance in identifying the politics lurking behind this and so many other publications relating to nutrition.[21]

I was interested to see how the food industry reacted to Professor Jim Mann's article published in the *British Medical Journal* describing the relationship between ingested sugars and body weight.[22] The Canadian Sugar Institute was quick to respond on their 'Health Professional' website—as one would predict. But in addition *Obesity Reviews* published a contrary view with the disclosures that 'corresponding author Dr. Allison has received consulting fees from Kraft Foods. The University of Alabama at Birmingham has received gifts and grants from multiple organizations including but not limited to The

Coca-Cola Company, PepsiCo, Red Bull and Kraft Foods.'[23]
A flurry of conflicting articles followed and in December
2013 *PloS Medicine* published a paper that examined the role
of financial conflicts of interest in relation to studies linking
sugar-sweetened beverages (SSBs) and weight gain. They found
that in the reviews conducted by authors who declared no
conflict of interest, 83.3% thought that SSBs were a potential risk
factor for weight gain. In contrast the findings of 83.5% of the
papers written by authors declaring a conflict of interest thought
that there was insufficient information to support an association
between the two.[24]

In New Zealand the Food and Grocery Council (FGC) is an
industry lobby group headed by ex-National Party MP Katherine
Rich. Their website states that the FGC promotes the role the
industry plays in the health and nutrition of New Zealanders
in making better diet and lifestyle choices (that is, it is a matter
of personal responsibility). When Coca-Cola announced a
four-point plan to counter obesity it was lauded by the FGC (and
panned by public health advocates) and the organization opposed
the move to follow Australia with a clear food labeling system.
What is curious is that Rich was also appointed to the board of
a supposedly neutral government body—the Health Promotion
Agency. This appointment raises the question of undue corporate influence on governmental policymaking, but the story in
this case gets murkier as it appears that Rich was also involved in
the denigration of public health specialists and academics via the
right-wing blogger Whale Oil. With luck, the response to this and
other revelations in Nicky Hager's book *Dirty Politics* will be a
re-examination of the appointment of those with vested interests
to advisory positions.[25]

Grabbing land and water

While the ingredients for processed foods are cheap, they aren't free. One way to keep costs low is to base production in countries where land, labor, and even water are inexpensive. In this modern version of colonization, small-scale food production for the local market is replaced by growing food as a commodity for first world countries. To make cheap processed food you need palm oil and sugar cane. A lot of attention has been paid to high-fructose corn syrup and the possibility that as a sweetener it is particularly harmful. But reliance on sucrose comes with another set of problems—not the least being, where do you get the land to grow the sugar cane (or beets)? Oxfam's Behind the Brands campaign found that globally 31 million hectares of land (an area the size of Italy) is devoted to growing sugar and the demand is predicted to grow by 25% by 2020. Land grabbing becomes a real possibility. For example, Oxfam describes a small community from the Sirinhaem Estuary in Brazil who were harassed by the private militia of the sugar company Trapiche, and eventually evicted by law so that Trapiche could use their land to grow sugar cane for Coca-Cola and Pepsi.

Even without the force that appears to have been used in the Sirinhaem Estuary case there is real cause for concern for small-scale farmers in developing countries. Oxfam reports that since 2000, 33 million hectares globally have been sold to foreign investors. Most of this is to produce food for export, thereby increasing food insecurity and hunger for the local populations. The three big players in this market—Associated British Foods (the world's second largest sugar producer), Coca-Cola, and Pepsi (major sugar consumers)—don't seem to have policies that control their supply chains and ensure that land is acquired ethically.[26] This is common. Fonterra imports annually 1.3 million tons of palm kernel expeller, a co-product of palm oil production, to feed dairy herds. The dairy co-operative buys it from the world's largest palm oil trader, Wilmar International, who in turn buys it from third parties so there is no way of ensuring that the palm oil Fonterra buys is ethically sourced. In addition, the destruction of rain forests to grow palms for oil production is a significant factor in greenhouse gas production.[27]

Commodification of food production by multinational companies leads to the loss of food sovereignty and often to the transfer of resources from areas of scarcity to rich countries that are already well supplied. Bottled water is an egregious example with water from countries where clean drinking water is in short supply going to first world countries where it's safe to drink straight from the tap. In southern Kerala, in India, thousands of villagers abandoned their orchards and gardens following the opening of a Coca-Cola bottling plant in 1999. Coca-Cola admitted to taking up to 600,000 liters of water a day from the aquifer (local protesters put the figure at 1 million liters) in a region where the small annual rainfall meant the opportunities for replenishment were low. In addition, waste from the bottling plant was being distributed as 'fertilizer,' presumably on the basis of high phosphate levels but testing also revealed toxic levels of cadmium and lead.

Corporate social responsibility?

When the food industry is accused of fueling the obesity epidemic their standard response is to say they are just meeting customer demand. Lately, either because of consumer demand or, more likely, scrutiny from anti-obesity campaigners, companies like McDonald's have been giving their customers a 'choice' of fruit and salads as well as soft drink and fries. The menu was introduced with great fanfare, but when challenged to demonstrate that sales of fries and burgers had dropped as a result the company declined. The sales didn't, and insiders tell me the salads have been a flop.

In 2013 Coca-Cola launched a campaign in New Zealand and Australia which not only acknowledged the problem of obesity, but hinted at their having a role in this. They are correct of course.[28] Coca-Cola listed the five steps they were taking to reduce obesity. To be successful their efforts would have to result in a decrease in the sales of sugar-sweetened drinks but they described the predictable combination of more choice of sizes and diet drinks (with the potential therefore to increase market share), deflection of attention to physical activity, and a promise to 'provide more transparent nutritional information in more places.' When the head of Coke New Zealand was asked if they would stop the sale of giant soft drink containers (single servings containing 44 teaspoons of sugar) in movie theaters he said *no*. In November 2013 the head of Coke Europe agreed that this should happen but as of November 2015 nothing's changed.

Disney has also acknowledged the obesity epidemic, promising not to allow the use of its characters to promote the sale of junk food to kids . . . but made an exception for food marketed during Halloween, Valentine's Day, Easter, or other special occasions. Christmas and these other special occasions account for 25% of their candy sales. Nestlé claims it doesn't market confectionery to children but made an exception for a line of Girl Scout–themed Crunch candy bars. These and other examples are listed on the 'Wall of Shame' of the Food Marketing Workgroup website (foodmarketing.org).

Michelle Simon, writing for Huff Post Business, targets McDonald's for failed promises to show corporate responsibility in the US. In 2002 McDonald's used beef tallow in its cooking oil while saying it was 100% vegetable oil. The case was settled for US$10 million. In the same year the company made a public promise to remove trans-fats from its cooking oil within six months. When it didn't follow through (or tell anyone it had failed to do so) they were found guilty of fraud and fined US$8.5 million. They also found a tricky workaround to avoid the San Francisco board of supervisors ruling that give-away toys could only be sold with healthy Happy Meals. Instead of changing the meals to make them healthier, McDonald's charged a pathetic 10 cents for the inclusion of the toy. Despite this history there was great excitement when McDonald's recently announced it was going to scrap soft drinks from its Happy Meals, with endorsement from Bill Clinton's Alliance for a Healthier Generation. Simon's skepticism led her to dig deeper and the real story is that they will only *promote* healthy drinks, but you can still choose the soft drink. She also describes the reality when it comes to the provision of healthy alternatives to fries—a move much lauded a year or so ago. It appears 80% of McDonald's outlets are owned by cash-strapped franchisees over which McDonald's has little control. These small businesses are 'encouraged' to provide a choice of side salad, fruit, or vegetable as an alternative at no extra cost, but in practice they don't because fries are cheaper and easier to prepare.[29]

As tobacco companies did 50 years ago, the fast food industry maintains its influence by spending money in high places.

The American Beverage Association, through its organization the Foundation for a Healthy America, gave $10 million to The Children's Hospital of Philadelphia at a time when the city of Philadelphia was considering a soda tax.[30] The American Dietetic Association and the British Nutrition Foundation are both generously supported by junk food and soft drink companies. Stephen Blair, a prominent publisher on the benefits of physical activity, admits to taking millions from Coca-Cola to fund his research. And Nestlé and Coca-Cola both paid to secure seats on the global policy board of WHO.[31]

Can we partner up with industry?

Striking a deal with industry is attractive—they have the might after all; if they apply their skills and resources in a manner that helps rather than harms, progress will surely be made. The million dollar question is 'Can we trust them?' Those who remember how the tobacco industry behaved when cigarette smoking was found to be harmful are inclined to say no. In 2013 the *British Medical Journal* hosted a debate asking 'Can we leave industry to lead efforts to improve population health?' Derek Yach, director of the Vitality Institute and one-time Pepsi employee, wrote in favor of the moot, giving examples such as Unilever removing salt from its products and Kraft taking out trans-fats. But even he didn't think it was likely that industry would take the lead.[32] David Stuckler and Marion Nestle wrote in opposition, making the point that there is a conflict of interest for companies that profit by selling the products we need to eat less of.[33] It's also hard to believe that industry is capable of socially responsible behavior when the self-governing bodies don't have the clout to ensure their members behave. For example, in 2010, the Hungry Jack's burger chain was exposed for ignoring Australia's industry-regulated advertising codes for children. They ran a *Simpsons*-themed advertisement for chicken nuggets that were found (after a complaint) to be too high in fat. The ad was banned but the company went on to run it a further 300 times.[34]

For any initiative intending to improve health at the cost of removing a market edge, adherence would require that this be applied across the board, that is, all companies would play by the rules. In 2005 Walmart launched a sustainability campaign which included a change in packaging to reduce landfill waste. The result was a sudden drop in sales as their competitors continued using the packaging that had been developed in response to shopper preferences. The new Walmart packaging was ditched. Free marketeers will say that when customers decide that green packaging is a priority for them, industry will evolve to match the demand . . . and that when society starts to demand healthy food, junk food will disappear. But how long would we have had to wait for the public to demand seatbelts, or restrictions on smoking in public places?

When Sarah Thomson (the CEO of Diabetes New Zealand) and I set up FOE (Fight the Obesity Epidemic) I decided not to blame industry, but rather to see their actions as the predictable consequence of a market-driven economy with insufficient rules to protect the population. But much of this profit-driven behavior is unethical in the same way the behavior of tobacco manufacturers has been, and continues to be. For decades the tobacco industry fought the science linking tobacco with lung cancer and vascular disease and the producers of sugar-sweetened beverages are just as fierce in their protestations that these products, for which there are no nutritional benefits, do no harm. As awareness of the harm related to tobacco increased, manufacturers shifted their focus to developing countries in an effort to milk the cash cow just a little longer. The food industry is following suit. As the markets for junk food become saturated, vulnerable communities in developing countries are being targeted to maintain sales. Hershey built a US$250 million plant in Malaysia in order to sell Hershey's chocolate throughout Asia. It already has a plant in China, which has reached capacity, and the company anticipated international sales of US$1 billion by the end of 2014.[35]

So does the food industry have a role in the genesis of the obesity epidemic? The answer is yes. They produce and promote the energy-dense foods of which we eat too much. More interesting is the question of whether they have a role in ending the obesity epidemic. Food producers say they do, but in so many ways their behavior mimics that of the tobacco industry so I don't trust them. At least, not yet.

The environmental factors promoting obesity are omnipresent but they don't affect us equally. Social factors like wealth and education may be as important as genes in determining our susceptibility to an adverse environment but obesity can influence our socio-economic status too. It's a chicken and egg thing.

8

How the overweight are stigmatized

If governments are to make progress with reducing obesity rates they need to be a lot more explicit about the association of obesity with social status and the effect of stigmatization on obese people. Obesity is already distributed unevenly across social groups, with poorer people more badly affected, and I fear governments are contributing to this inequality with their determination to make this an issue of personal responsibility.

Why is it that obesity and poverty track together? Poverty can cause obesity if healthy food is too expensive and obesity can cause poverty if earning potential is reduced through illness. A common cause for both could be low educational attainment (although some of the most clever and successful people I know are obese). Almost certainly, all three of these phenomena play a part. Speaking at a recent public health conference, I said the way health professionals currently treat obesity contravenes the

Hippocratic Oath of 'do no harm.' I'm particularly concerned by the ways in which obesity causes poverty and obese individuals are stigmatized.

How does poverty contribute to obesity?

Obesity rates have increased across all races, all levels of education, and all levels of income. The data from the National Health and Nutrition Examination Survey in the United States were used to compare obesity rates in boys and girls across two periods of time, from 1988 to 1994 and from 2005 to 2008. For wealthy boys the obesity rate went from 6.5% to 11.9%. For the poorest boys, the rate went from 12.5% to 21.1%.[1] Because the percentage of the US population in poverty has also increased, there has been an exaggerated effect on the numbers of people obese. In 1973 poverty affected 11.1% of the US population and in 2010 that figure was 15.2%.[2] Compounding the story further is the issue of ethnicity in relation to both predispositions to obesity and to poverty. In New Zealand overall child poverty rates are also about 15% but the ethnic variation is remarkable. Using a questionnaire of 'things that a family had to do without' to measure deprivation, 51% of Pacific Island children under the age of 17 were assessed as highly deprived. For Maori the figure is 39% and for European children it is 15%.[3] Changes in the ethnic make-up of populations over time will therefore also affect obesity rates.

It is easy to attribute variations in obesity rates between ethnicities to different cultural norms. In New Zealand food plays a large part in gatherings of Pasifika people but feasting is only part of the story. A study of almost 2,500 Pacific Island adolescents as part of the Obesity Prevention in Communities (OPIC) project found socio-environmental factors associated with poverty were more important than cultural factors in determining whether a Pacific student was obese or not. They identified lifestyle differences between the families earning a low income and those who were more financially secure. Obese students were more likely to live in households where no one was home during the day and they were less likely to eat breakfast, or lunch, than the normal weight students. Typically, large families were reliant on low wages, with shift work being a common form of employment; a shared evening meal was a rare event. Mothers working long hours didn't have time to cook so they would regularly eat takeaways (particularly fish and chips). Normal weight students included fruit and vegetables in the description of their diet; the overweight students talked about sausages (and no vegetables). In the qualitative part of this survey it was clear that everyone knew what healthy food was, and that they should be eating it— but they couldn't afford to. The imperative to buy white bread instead of wholegrain was based on cost—89 cents a loaf for white and up to NZ$5 for wholegrain.[4]

Access to unhealthy food via fast food outlets and convenience stores is also linked to decile rating. A survey throughout New Zealand found travel distances to fast food outlets were at least twice as far in the wealthy neighborhoods when compared to the most deprived neighborhoods.[5] But the story gets complicated when it comes to supermarkets. In public health literature big stores are assumed to provide access to healthy food but they are also the source of most unhealthy food too. The New Zealand survey found good access to supermarkets in poor neighborhoods and another from the UK found the same thing—the most deprived neighborhoods actually had the best access to grocery stores selling fresh produce.[6] This in part reflects the higher population density of poorer urban environments but it does suggest that lifestyles might be driving the demand for fast food rather than the other way around. The same researchers found a higher density of alcohol retail outlets in poor areas when compared to wealthy.

One of the reasons the issue of food supply and social demographics is so difficult to unravel is that the whole phenomenon of urbanization is evolving. In the 1950s the term 'white flight' was used to describe the abandonment of the inner city by the middle classes and their subsequent colonization of the suburbs. Today, throughout the world, the upper and middle classes are returning to the inner cities and the poor, immigrant, and minority populations are being forced to settle in the suburbs and rural towns. When you add in factors such as urban versus rural and high- or low-minority population estimates you do find that in low-density urban areas it is the high-poverty and/or high-minority groups who have the lowest access to grocery stores and supermarkets and the highest access to fast food outlets.[7] The complexity of this issue does, however, suggest that policy interventions with regard to the density of food outlets might be better aimed at restricting unhealthy food vendors in specific environments (around schools for example) or across the board, rather than a targeted approach for low-decile areas—given that some of our assumptions about 'food deserts' and 'food swamps' appear to be incorrect.

Perhaps, though, it's just the cost of food that matters? The cost per calorie is clearly much higher for fruit and vegetables than energy-dense processed food and the latter therefore represents better value for money. A recent estimate from the US puts the cost per megajoule for potato chips at 20 cents, while the cost for carrots is 95 cents. Even if meeting calorie demands isn't the main issue, the fact that the price of fresh fruit and vegetables has risen sharply in relation to the CPI—and even more so in comparison to sweets and soft drinks—will have an effect on the food we buy. Raising the price of cigarettes over the years has been an effective way of reducing consumption and many cafeteria studies have shown that food choice is very price sensitive. Kelly Brownell, professor of public policy at Duke University, and others performed a systematic review of the price elasticity of food and found it varied depending on the type of food. Price had the greatest influence on the choices people made when they were selecting soft drinks, juice, meat, takeaway food, and when dining out. The expectation is that price sensitivity would be greater for those with less discretionary income for whom value for money is likely to be more important. This data indicated that if soft drink prices increased by 10%, then sales would drop by 8–10%.[8] We now have seen this in action with Mexico, which introduced a sugar tax on soft drinks in 2014. After 12 months of a 10% tax, sales fell by 6% overall and by 9% in low-income families. In subsequent months there was a 12% drop overall and a 17% drop for poorer families.[9] The role of food may also differ between poor and wealthy families. Food may function as a reward or treat for low-income families, taking the place of more expensive presents or holidays. The bottom line is that poorer families spend less per capita on food than well-off families and what they buy is cheaper and higher in calories.[10]

An alternative explanation for the link between poverty and food choices is provided by researchers who believe there are 'deeply rooted, neuro-endocrine responses to economic insecurity' that promote weight gain. In a paper entitled 'Why the poor get fat: weight gain and economic insecurity' the authors describe how over a 12-year period a 50% drop in annual income is associated with a 5 pound weight gain over and above the 21 pounds gained by the average American male. This is no more than an association but they offer a novel explanation that roughly says that eating more in the face of insecurity is a primitive biological response that we haven't quite lost.[11] Such a response would provide justification for panic or comfort eating. It's an interesting idea—appetite is controlled by the hypothalamus where the oldest, most primitive behaviors derive, and one can see that income insecurity (and perhaps other forms of threat) rather than income itself may well be a stimulus to increase fat reserves.

What about the possibility of a common mechanism for both poverty and obesity? People with intellectual impairment are likely to be poor and unable to make appropriate food choices or to cook for themselves, and those suffering from mental illness may have their problems exacerbated by treatment with potent appetite-stimulating anti-psychotic medication. But what about the role of education, or lack of, as a cause of both poverty and obesity? I spoke at a food bank conference once and was told food banks couldn't give out raw ingredients because most of the users of the service didn't know how to cook (nor did they have pots or pans).

But ability to cook doesn't closely track with poverty. In the nineteenth century the servant classes cooked for the wealthy. By halfway through the next century, middle-class women were home-based, doing cordon bleu courses or at least their own preserving in addition to preparing the family meals. Girls were taught to cook and sew at intermediate school (I'm a product of this era and spent the weekend pickling beetroot and making lemon curd). Boys were taught woodwork and metalwork and of course most men couldn't cook—their role was as income earner. From that time onwards the increased participation of women in the workforce, urbanization, access to preprepared meals, increasing wealth as well as increasing poverty have resulted in many individuals no longer having the skills, or the time—or even the need—to cook. For many, cooking has become a hobby, or a form of television entertainment, but I suspect that 'not knowing how to cook' is prevalent among young wealthy urbanites.

Some academics make the point that it's actually a web of conditions that link low income and poor health, that not only obesity but many forms of illness translate into premature death as a result of low income. One set of researchers calculated that 25% of all deaths occurring in Virginia between 1996 and 2002 would have been averted if the mortality rate matched that of the five most affluent counties.[12] The coexistence of poverty, low education and poor health is demonstrated by the statistic that in the United States apparently 50% of all male deaths and 40% of all female deaths between the ages of 25 and 64 would not occur if everyone attained the mortality rates of college graduates.[13] While it seems unlikely that there is a simple causal link between low education levels and poor health, effort applied to education may well be more effective than delivering more healthcare or even targeted health information as a means of improving health outcomes—including obesity.

How does obesity contribute to poverty?

Chronic diseases impoverish both the individual and society. If you develop diabetes as part of the metabolic syndrome you are likely to need a raft of medications to measure and treat elevated blood sugar, hypertension, and abnormal lipids. It would not be unusual to have a dozen items on a prescription list. If you live in Chennai, India, you might have to spend a quarter of your income on diabetes care.[14] If you are an airline pilot, or work on a deep-sea oil rig, or drive a heavy freight vehicle and require insulin therapy, you will lose your job. Insurance companies will often charge higher premiums for obese individuals (especially life insurance) and if you are an obese person flying Samoan Airlines, you will be charged a higher ticket price. In addition, the combination of unemployment and premature death deprives families of resources that could be used for investment.

Lower employment means that obese people pay less tax and collect more unemployment and sickness benefits. But they also die, on average, eight years earlier than non-obese people and as with cigarette smokers this could be viewed as a fiscal advantage as obese people don't collect the old-age pension for as long. Woodward and Blakely in their overview of life and death in New Zealand, *The Healthy Country?*, considered whether the effect of obesity was strong enough to reverse the inexorable increase in longevity for the population and thought that this was unlikely. What they do predict, however, is an expansion of chronic illness with obese individuals experiencing more years of disability during their foreshortened life.[15] To estimate the overall economic impact of obesity, sophisticated models take into account both direct medical costs and lost productivity. The prediction is for 65 million more obese adults in the US and 11 million more obese adults in the UK by 2030. Totalling up the costs related to diabetes, cancer, heart disease, stroke and adding to this the quality-adjusted life years lost results in additional costs of $48–66 billion a year in the US and £1.9–2 billion a year in the UK.[16] A similar study in New Zealand estimated the combined costs of healthcare expenditure and productivity loss to be about NZ$800 million (more or less depending on the model used) with the healthcare costs alone amounting to 4.4% of the health budget. About half of the costs related to type 2 diabetes.[17]

But even for obese individuals who are well and capable of working, the odds are stacked against them attaining wealth. British research showed that the probability of being in employment was significantly lower (up to 25%) for obese people than non-obese and that this was the same for men and women. This is the result of prejudice not disability.

How we discriminate on the basis of weight (and what this does)

The hidden costs of obesity are those that result from discrimination rather than physical impairment. Rebecca Puhl is a senior scientist and deputy director at the Rudd Center for Food Policy and Obesity at Yale University and an expert on discrimination against obese individuals. Her comprehensive (and depressing) review of the subject provides many explanations for an inverse relationship between weight and wealth.[18] The data from experimental work along with that from literature searches and meta-analyses demonstrate that bias on the basis of weight is pervasive, usually stronger than that on the basis of ethnicity, and increasing. Appallingly, health professionals—especially those who work in the field of weight management—are among the worst offenders. Large cross-sectional studies show that not only is obesity associated with lower employment but also that within the workforce there is a wage penalty associated with being overweight. In a survey using data from the National Longitudinal Survey of Youth (with a total of 25,843 participants) an increase of 64 pounds above average weight in white women was associated with a 9% decrease in wages, which was approximately equivalent to 1.5 years of education or three years of work experience.[19] These relationships held true for black women (less marked) and also for men, with severely obese men earning 19.6% less than average and black men 3.5% less than average.[20]

Backing up the cross-sectional surveys are a great many experiments that demonstrate a causal relationship between employment and weight. In some, actors wore padded clothing to mimic obesity and in others, cartoons or mock photographs were used and, irrespective of qualifications or work experience, the chances of being employed are lower if you are overweight or obese. Many additional studies indicate the reason for this is that obese people are viewed as being less conscientious, less agreeable, less emotionally stable, and less extroverted than their normal weight counterparts. Needless to say, other studies which measure individual personality traits disprove these associations. Over and above the financial impact of this discrimination in the workplace is the emotional impact of pejorative comments and being the target of derogatory humour. A survey of overweight and obese women found that 54% reported weight stigma from colleagues or co-workers and 43% from their employer or supervisors.[21]

What's particularly tragic is the impact of prejudice on obese children and young adults, and the fact that this appears to be increasing. The psychologist Professor Janet Latner and Albert Stunkard (of twin studies fame) tested the attitudes of fifth and sixth graders from different schools towards a range of physical characteristics using a survey first conducted in 1961, and then compared their results with the original survey.[22] The children were provided with a series of cards on which were sketched other children and they were asked to select the person they most wanted for a friend. They were asked to do this one card at a time until all the cards were gone. The cartoon child was variously shown as having no distinguishing features; or having a disfigured face; or missing a hand. One was shown with crutches and another had a wheelchair. Another was obese. In both 1961 and 2001 the child with no remarkable features was the most favoured friend and the obese child was the least favoured. There was a gender difference with girls having more of an aversion to impaired appearance (ranking the disfigured child low) and boys to impaired performance (ranking the children with crutches or the wheelchair low), but both ranked the obese child last. Between 1961 and 2001 the middle order of the disfigured and disabled children changed somewhat but the spread between the top-ranked child and bottom-ranked actually increased over that time. What interests me most is the fact that obese children participating in the study didn't differ from their peers in the way they ranked the choices.

British psychologist Andy Hill conducted experiments with 9-year-olds using silhouette figures of either slim or overweight boys and girls. On testing he found the children associated the overweight figure with poor social functioning, impaired academic success, unhealthy eating and low levels of fitness.[23] Hill is an expert on adolescents and young adults and says that at this age friendships are the most important thing in a child's life and that these are essential for normal development—probably more so than parental influence. In another study of friendship, he asked children to list the names of other children that they considered to be their friends. They then looked at to what extent these matched up (ideally the lists would be reciprocal) and drew maps of the linkages. The resulting diagram was a nest with the center consisting of the children who had lots of friends who mostly liked them back and around the perimeter were the kids who had only one friend, who sometimes did not reciprocate the friendship. The researchers had also graded the children according to weight and, lo and behold, the children with few or no reciprocated friendships were obese. Sadly this prejudice develops very early. In an experiment with kindergarten-aged children 86% expressed an aversion to photographs of overweight children.[24] The most alarming evidence of stigmatization comes from a study of college students, which recorded the financial support they received from their family as well as their weight, and it could be seen that parents are more likely to lend money to their slim children compared to their overweight daughters.[25]

It is no surprise then to find that overweight people are less likely to be offered a job, to be promoted, or to marry when compared to their slim colleagues. In addition to this, significantly overweight people experience awful prejudice when out in public—people peer into their supermarket trolleys and make comments on the contents; derisory remarks are muttered if they dare to eat an ice cream in public; and air travel is fraught with opportunities for embarrassment. I am ashamed to say that doctors contribute significantly to the stigmatization and as a result obese people are reluctant to attend appointments for any but the most urgent of problems. This means they miss out on routine screening such as cervical smear tests and mammograms and they often present much later in an illness than they should. This is compounded by the fact that it is difficult to make a diagnosis on the basis of physical examination; many routine tests such as ultrasound and even X-rays are difficult to interpret and some, like MRI scans, may be ruled out if the patient is unable to fit through the scanner. As a result obese people are sometimes perilously ill without this being very apparent. I remember some years ago an obese woman coming to the emergency department of the hospital where I was a consultant physician and receiving a call from the registrar who was embarrassed because she was having difficulty persuading the patient to have a blood test or to allow an intravenous line to be inserted. I came over to help and realized that although she appeared reasonably well the woman was confused because of sepsis and deteriorating fast. We called for assistance from the intensive care unit staff but she had a cardiac arrest before they arrived. She was resuscitated and later taken to surgery to remove a large area of infected abdominal wall that wouldn't have been visible to the patient because of her weight. Sadly she died a few days later.

The drivers of obesity stigma

At the core of anti-obesity prejudice is the belief that individuals can control their weight and that obese people choose not to. In studies conducted with US and Australian university students a correlation can be seen between attitudes of 'disgust' towards a range of social groups and the perception of control associated with the membership of that group. For example, mental illness didn't rate highly on the scale of disgust nor was it seen as a condition over which individuals had great control. At the other end of the scale, drug addicts and smokers were given the highest score on the disgust scale and assessed as having a high degree of perceived control over their situation. We can debate the validity of these perceptions but the interest is in the linear association between disgust and control. Obese individuals were rated next after smokers and only slightly ahead of politicians on the disgust scale and were thought to have a reasonably high degree of control over their situation. The author of this paper wondered about the origin of the emotion of disgust in relation to obesity and suggested that there was a moralization element—that opting to be fat when the ideal is for slim transgressed some moral code.[26] More support for the notion of control as a driver of anti-obesity stigma comes from an experiment in which psychology students were surveyed to measure the extent of 'anti-fat prejudice' before and after a tutorial on obesity. For those who learned about diet and exercise as a means of dealing with obesity the prejudice measure didn't change. For those who took part in a tutorial on geno-environmental causes of obesity, the anti-fat prejudice rating dropped.[27]

We need to understand the potential for stigmatization alongside possible solutions to the obesity epidemic.[28] This is more than a moral or ethical consideration. Experience tells us that depending on the issue, either denormalization or destigmatization will be a more effective public health approach. Framing cigarette smoking as a bizarre behavior that's dangerous not only to smokers but also to close bystanders led to the progressive banning of smoking on planes, in movie theaters, hospitals, most workplaces, restaurants, and even bars. The sad sight of cold workers huddled outside on pavements looking for shelter while they smoke is about more than just protection of fellow workers. It is powerfully stigmatizing and, in conjunction with the very high cost of cigarettes, is credited with helping people quit smoking.

When AIDS was first identified and it became clear that a public health response was required, a similar, stigmatizing approach was taken. It was a disaster. The public panicked, those at risk of infection went into hiding, and engagement with programs to reduce infection was low. A major breakthrough occurred when the approach changed to one of normalization. I was a hospital doctor when AIDS was first recognized (we were all terrified of it) and can attest to the success of this change in tack, with the illness now viewed like any other treated in medical outpatient clinics. It's essential that we adopt a strategy of destigmatization in our public health approach to obesity. Not only because of the harm to individuals if we continue to consider it an issue of personal responsibility, but because this is the way to reduce the prevalence of obesity.

Many if not *most* of the things we do to reduce obesity currently fail the destigmatization test. Anything that emphasizes education and motivation of individuals certainly does so. Using a framework that divides up anti-obesity initiatives according to whether they are environmental or behavioral, and grades their potential for stigmatization as low, medium, or high, shows that environmental solutions such as taxation or restrictions on the placement of fast food restaurants have a low potential for stigmatization whereas endorsement of weight loss programs through the workplace depends on behavioral change, targets obese individuals and is highly stigmatizing. Even activities such as the provision of weight loss programs in primary care and increasing health education in school potentially increase prejudice by emphasizing personal choice.

The evidence of prejudice on the basis of body weight leading to psychological and physical ill has prompted some to argue that governments need to deal with weight discrimination in formal legislation.[29] I'm not sure legislating against discrimination in the workplace on the basis of body size (as has been suggested) is the right course of action but everyone needs to have greater awareness of anti-obesity prejudice. Before we berate individuals for failing to choose healthy food or lifestyles, the conditions to allow these choices will need to be optimized. If the default food environment is ready access (in terms of price as well as physical location) to healthy food then it is likely that there will be a marked reduction in those who make the effort to purchase unhealthy food. Similarly, when the default physical environment is one which favors cycling as the means to travel to work and school, you see many more people on bicycles than in cars—compare a city like Amsterdam with a car-oriented city like Auckland.

Improving our obesogenic environment requires an overarching nutrition strategy. Decisions made by trade and industry, by local councils, schools, transport authorities, and so forth should be tested for impact on population health with a particular emphasis on diet and exercise. Only governments can make this happen. But will they?

PART 3

What we can do about it

9

How governments can flick the switch

In Austria 99.9% of people permit their organs to be used after death but only 4.25% of Danes do. In both countries it's an issue of free choice, so what's different? It's possible Austrians are more generous than Danes, but a more likely explanation is the default which operates in each country. In Austria you need to opt out of organ donation and in Denmark you need to opt in. This simple piece of bureaucracy makes it easier or harder to do the right thing.[1]

Can we apply the same approach to the food environment? In a campaign in South Auckland the local diabetes team negotiated a deal with McDonald's to make the diet version of Sprite the default offering. Customers who wanted Sprite could still have the full sugar version, but they had to ask specifically. The result? A 17% reduction in sugar consumed. Think of the calorie reduction if they'd also agreed to do this with Coke.

Here's a slightly different example, courtesy of Boyd Swinburn, Professor of Population Nutrition and Global Health at the University of Auckland and director of the WHO Collaborating Centre for Obesity Prevention. New Zealanders eat potato chips by the ton, so reducing the fat content of chips would take a lot of calories out of the diet. To do this health officials could either persuade more people to choose low-fat chips, which drop chip calories by 30% for those people, or manufacturers could reduce the amount of fat in ordinary chips by an imperceptibly small amount. With the second option people wouldn't have to change their behavior, and vast numbers of calories would be stripped from the national diet without any sense of individual sacrifice.

Changing the default environment can support healthier choices in hundreds of ways but it takes a fundamental shift in thinking to see nutrition as an issue of societal responsibility. If obesity could be reduced by educating people to make sustained changes in behavior that would be fantastic. But it can't. Despite the great efforts of individuals the population is getting fatter and fatter. It's time to look at the ways in which governments can assist us to make healthy choices.

Will nudging do it?

Does government intervention mean regulation, or is there another way? Richard Thaler and Cass Sunstein, Chicago economists and co-authors of *Nudge*, argued that solving the public health problems created by the free market economy won't be achieved by regulation but by governments partnering up with industry. They define nudging as:

any aspect of the choice architecture [environment] that alters people's behavior in a predictable way without forbidding any options or significantly changing their economic incentives. To count as a nudge, the intervention must be easy and cheap to avoid.[2]

So any interference with the free market by external agencies is specifically excluded from 'nudging' by definition. It depends instead on industry players being good corporate citizens and innovating in ways to improve health outcomes. This approach is underpinned by the notion of 'libertarian paternalism' in which choices are offered in a manner likely to enhance wellbeing but the individual is still free to make a poor decision. As you might imagine, industrialists and politicians support any alternative to regulation and the British coalition government appointed Richard Thaler as an advisor on regulation issues. This was useful, I guess, in that it shifted emphasis away from the individual and identified that industry had a role to play in making us all healthier but it was part of a deregulatory thrust by the Cameron administration.

The concept of nudging spans a wide range of behaviors and law professor Robert Baldwin from the London School of Economics and Political Science divides nudging into three degrees. Typically first-degree nudging is the provision of simple information and reminders. Second-degree nudging introduces a bias by such things as opt-outs instead of opt-ins and changes to the physical environment—he gives the example of smoking areas being placed a long way from the work space to discourage smoking. Third-degree nudging is where manipulation of behavior occurs as a result of triggering emotional responses and includes subliminal advertising.[3]

149

Placing chocolate at a cut-rate price beside the till at the gas station is a second-degree nudge that increases the likelihood of you buying chocolate when you intended to just buy petrol. Thaler suggests these techniques can influence our decision-making for the better. Almost certainly they can. Health psychology professor Theresa Marteau says putting fruit beside the cash register in the cafeteria increased by 70% the amount of fruit school children bought at lunchtime. In another example shoppers bought more fruit and vegetables when there was marked space for these in supermarket trolleys. But, she says, regulation is much more effective.

In an effort to reduce hypertension and stroke, the British government entered nudging-type agreements with the food industry and promoted salt reduction via public health networks. Gateshead Council responded by conducting research showing that the local fish and chip shops were using flour shakers with up to 17 holes as salt dispensers and replaced these free of charge with ones that had only five holes. This and similar kinds of initiatives successfully reduced salt intake by 0.9 grams per person per day. The recommended upper limit is 5.7 grams a day. Meanwhile Finland and Japan decided to *regulate* the salt intake of food and this resulted in a reduction of 5 grams per person per day. Marteau argues that most examples of nudging aren't evaluated and they may in fact be very expensive methods of changing behavior. Nor are successful initiatives likely to be sustained without the evidence that supports change. Even worse, reliance on these soft options delays the introduction of regulation-based changes predicted to be much more effective.[4] Geof Rayner, a former head of the UK Public Health Association, and Tim Lang, the first professor of food policy in the UK, are co-authors of

Ecological Public Health and are even more damning of nudging as an approach and suggest that it's a collusion between state and corporations to hoodwink consumers.[5]

But I think the real issue is the unconscious nature of third degree nudging as described by Baldwin. While these may be commonly used techniques in the world of marketing, should governments be engaging in the same unethical behavior? I think the public expect efforts to change our environment to be overt so that we can rationally debate them. In considering whether a government should engage in nudging, Baldwin suggests that a choice needs to be made; is the autonomy of targeted individuals to be respected and openly worked with, or reduced and their decision-making to be nudged by stealth?

Do governments have a mandate to intervene in the free market for food?

If individuals can't do it by themselves, and industry is incapable of effective self-regulation, should governments intervene? Economic purists argue there has to be evidence of market failure to justify interference with the laws of supply and demand which underpin the commercial world. Government intervention should be considered only if conditions meet one of the criteria of market failure.[6]

The first criteria is skewing of the market by 'externalities'. This refers to an individual making a conscious decision which results in a bad outcome, the cost of which is borne by someone else. Ideally, only you should suffer the consequences of your bad decisions. If, for example, you want to sky-dive or climb

151

mountains the risks associated with those activities (dying) fall on you. With obesity a person may choose to eat an unhealthy diet but if they develop obesity-related disease the costs of this are borne by society as well as that individual, and if the financial costs are too high, the government would have grounds to intervene. It is easy to make this case. An estimate of the global cost of obesity to individuals is 36 million disability-adjusted life years (DALYs) but there are also direct medical costs for the state.[7] A recent paper from the *Journal of Health Economics* attributes 20.8% of medical costs in the United States to obesity.[8] Added to this are the indirect costs of a reduced tax take for those who are on sick leave or out of work and the impact of reduced income on the family of an obese individual. In 2010 diabetes alone cost the global economy US$500 billion.[9] The economic imperative for intervention in the market is powerful.

The second version of market failure occurs when 'imperfect information' perverts our ability to make a reasoned decision. Do most people know enough about nutrition to choose one food over another? The furious debate on Twitter (#paleo, #futureoffoods) at the moment about whether animal fat is bad or good suggests not. Imperfect information certainly applies to confusing food labeling on processed foods. How on earth do shoppers decide if these products made from artificial ingredients are healthy? In addition to price, consumers would like to know what country food comes from and, for many, whether animal farming practices are humane, or if the food is the product of genetic engineering. Left to the manufacturers, they will add information labels if they confer a sales advantage but not otherwise. Governments seem modestly interested in tackling food labels but the fact that the food industry has lobbied so hard to avoid these suggests that imperfect information works in their favor and may well be skewing the supply and demand equation.

The third category is 'time-inconsistent preferences', which often result in satisfying short-term goals over longer-term ones. I would have thought this was a constant feature of everyday life but in this context it could refer to planning to cook a healthy meal but succumbing to the temptation to eat from the junk food outlets that you pass on the way home. A way of correcting for this would be to ensure that healthy food was available in all places where unhealthy food is sold. Choosing to drive your car to work instead of taking public transport might also fit into this category.

I'm most interested in the fourth category of 'demerit goods,' meaning products like alcohol and tobacco and activities such as gambling which are dangerous or unhealthy. Governments are bound to protect vulnerable individuals from the market forces of supply and demand for these goods and services. With regard to obesity, foods which are energy dense and without nutritional value (apart from calories) are demerit goods. As to vulnerable individuals, the emphasis is appropriately on children and adolescents because they demonstrate poor appreciation of the long-term consequences of their decisions, haven't developed self-management skills, and peer pressure (by other bad decision-makers) often exceeds that of parents. Tobacco companies worked that out decades ago, and their marketing strategies ignore older adults in favor of 16- and 17-year-olds, knowing that sufficient numbers will become addicted to smoking and so provide them with a lifelong customer. Parents know this and have been pushing hard for governments to restrict junk food advertising but, as well as children, anyone with an inherited predisposition towards obesity deserves protection.

153

Politicians are motivated to take actions that will increase the chance of election. This requires correctly identifying the public mood for change as well as keeping in good with powerful lobbyists who provide funding and voter support if policies are favorable to their interests. While most people support restrictions on the marketing of junk food and soft drinks, the libertarian cry, supported by those with a vested interest in maintaining an unregulated market, remains strong. Developing policy in such a highly charged environment isn't straightforward.

In December 2007 the New Zealand Labour government introduced to Parliament a revised version of the Public Health Act. A small clause allowed the Director General of Health to introduce regulations if, after a two-year trial, industry failed to live up to agreed codes of conduct with regard to non-communicable disease risks. When the Bill had its first reading in the House I remember the opposition health spokesperson, Tony Ryall, responding hysterically. He warned of the government restricting what food could be sold in schools and workplaces, preventing sponsorship of sporting activities by food and drink manufacturers and even (absurdly) limiting the sale of fish and chips to adults only. This Act disappeared with the change in government and, eight years on, the prediction with regard to the sale of fish and chips (New Zealand's favorite takeaway) remains outlandish but the other examples are now mainstream recommendations.

Research can now help policymakers understand what is and isn't likely to be acceptable in the way of regulation. For example, a group of individuals and focus groups interviewed by Dutch researchers believed strongly that people are responsible for their own choice of food and that freedom of choice is a great good that should be preserved. They felt that encouragement of good choices was better than discouragement of bad choices, that increasing the accessibility of healthy foods was more fair than restricting access to unhealthy foods, and they didn't support education campaigns designed to discourage people from eating poorly as they didn't think they would work. They were strongly in favor of clear food labels.[10]

So while scientific evidence indicates that behavior is no more than a predictable biological response to a set of environmental stimuli, and if individuals have a strong need to maintain a belief that they are sentient beings with control over their lives, then solutions to the obesity epidemic that restrict choice are going to be resisted—at least initially. In addition, public perception of what's likely to be effective or not isn't necessarily correct and will vary from one society to another and over time. Think of the change in attitudes to the wearing of seatbelts and to smoking in public places. Policymakers and politicians need to understand local belief systems in order to anticipate which interventions will be seen as acceptable and also which are likely to cause resistance and fail.

Where is the evidence?

In 2001 when I was president of the New Zealand Society for the Study of Diabetes and Sarah Thomson was CEO of Diabetes New Zealand we formed FOE (Fight the Obesity Epidemic) to raise awareness of obesity as a problem. We had the figures showing how common obesity was and how it was changing over time, and the back-up of plenty of studies demonstrating the failure of dieting and health promotion. But there was little evidence as to the causes or likely effective interventions. The medical world was (and still is) obsessed with evidence-based medicine and the randomized, placebo-controlled, double-blind trial as the way to determine this. Politicians opposed to or fearful of regulation were quick to point to a lack of evidence as justification for inaction. But this situation is changing.

Evidence gathering in public health is a different exercise to that undertaken by pharmaceutical companies seeking FDA-approval for a new drug. Instead of using randomized, placebo-controlled trials, public health initiatives can be evaluated in other ways. For example, the Minnesota Heart Health Program, a community-based intervention trial, collected outcome data demonstrating the *ineffectiveness* of health promotion as a way of reducing BMI in the local population.[11] You wouldn't know this from the number of times the same solutions have been suggested over the subsequent decades and even as I write this the government is suggesting such a program, Healthy Families, as New Zealand's solution to the obesity epidemic. It is modelled on a program from the State of Victoria, Australia, where children in the targeted communities lost a kilogram in weight and were fitter as a result of their participation. But this approach has already been shown not to work for Maori and Pacific Island children. Sadly, ignoring evidence is a long-standing problem in the scientific world.

I've just learned the term 'population science' from Nick Wareham, a British geneticist who believes that observing natural experiments in society is the way to accumulate evidence to tell us which interventions are worth replicating. The example he gave was comparing the levels of physical activity of a town's inhabitants before and after introducing policies to encourage cycling. Another natural experiment was described by researchers at the University of California, Berkeley, looking at the effect of proximity of fast food outlets to schools. They studied 3 million ninth graders and found that if there was a fast food outlet within a tenth of a mile there were 5.2% more obese children in that school than if it was farther away. They calculated this on the basis of the children consuming between 30 and 100 extra calories a day, and the effect wore off once the distance had increased to a quarter of a mile (presumably the school kids couldn't be bothered to walk farther).[12]

The sort of data already collected by governments or the agencies they fund could guide public health interventions. So much of this valuable material is never analyzed and goes to waste. Only government agencies are going to collect measurements of BMI for different sub-sets of the population along with the intermediate markers of obesity such as nutritional and physical activity surveys, public transport usage, levels of poverty and food disappearance data. Determining how much a population is consuming is extraordinarily difficult and calculating the amount of food that's produced (and disappears) is as close as you can get. It includes food that's wasted but assuming that this doesn't change significantly the food disappearance data provides useful information about change in calorie consumption over time.

Historical evidence from other public health interventions is another source of information governments could be looking at. The obvious example is the campaign to first increase, and then to reduce, smoking. Federal taxation in the US began with tobacco products as a revenue collecting exercise to cover the costs of the Civil, then the Spanish American, War. In 1880, 50% of the tax revenue came from chewing and smoking pipe tobacco, 40% from

cigars, and only 2% from cigarettes. In 1920 there were almost
no cigarette smokers and the excise tax dropped from $1.75 to
50 cents for a thousand cigarettes. Soldiers received free cigarettes during the First World War and by 1935, 50% of American
men smoked. The first reports of the addictive nature of nicotine
appeared in 1942, the link with lung cancer was confirmed in the
1950s, and by 1963 there were 3,000 published articles describing
the adverse health effects of smoking. From that time onwards
the prevalence of smoking in the US fell steadily. The US banned
cigarette advertisements in 1971 and the effectiveness of this
intervention was demonstrated when Ronald Reagan revoked the
ban in response to lobbying by industry. Tobacco sales went up
again so the bans were reintroduced. Now in the US, 26% of men
and 21% of women smoke and in New Zealand the latest census
has the smoking rate down at 15%.

Taxes are more effective than advertising bans. On the
economics of tobacco control, the World Bank reported that
increasing prices through taxation was the most cost-effective
measure for reducing cigarette consumption when compared to
non-fiscal measures or nicotine replacement therapy.[13] Others
reported that tax increases (they have to be high enough),
along with restrictions on access and bans on advertising, are
all cost-effective means of reducing alcohol consumption too.[14]
(Unlike prohibition which was a dismal failure.) It looks as if
these same measures will also work for junk food consumption.

When you don't have real-life examples to draw on theoret-
ical models can identify which interventions are likely to work
best. One example is the chronic disease prevention model,
comparing a range of interventions in Brazil, China, England,
India, Mexico, Russia, and South Africa. The DALYs saved and

the cost-effectiveness at 20 years and 50 years were calculated. The first finding (pretty obvious) is that in poor countries with low standards of healthcare to start with you get big improvements for relatively little cost, that if you want fast results for individuals you are better to target the high-risk population, but the best value for money comes from relatively inexpensive interventions that affect the entire population. Most cost-effective was regulating food advertising (750,000 life years saved), followed by fiscal measures such as taxes and subsidies (450,000), then food labeling, school-based interventions, physician counselling, worksite interventions, and lastly mass media campaigns (250,000).[15] Actually almost the same results were reported by Boyd Swinburn's group in 2006—restricting TV advertising saved 37,000 DALYs, targeted multi-faceted school-based programs saved 50, and walking school buses saved 30.[16] Guess which ones our governments are supporting.

Statistical modeling of taxation is now very sophisticated. A paper published in January 2014 from the National Bureau of Economic Research (NBER), a non-profit research organization, uses a structural quadratic almost ideal demand system (QAIDS) model. The authors compared taxing products (like soft drinks or snack foods) with taxing nutrients (sugar, fat, or salt). They applied a 20% tax in each example. With the nutrient model, the change in price is proportional to the amount of unhealthy ingredient. This sounds similar to the nutrient profiling model developed by Mike Rayner and his group in Oxford (see chapter seven).[17] This scores food, giving positive points for healthiness and negative points for unhealthiness, and was developed for food labeling. I heard Mike Rayner describing this model at a conference many years ago and remember that they scored the

159

food using this system and then tested it with a panel of dieticians to see if the scores lined up with their personal views of what was and wasn't 'healthy.' One controversial food was cheese which was deemed 'unhealthy' in Britain for some purpose or other but this was so counter to the ordinary public view that it attracted a lot of negative attention. Nutrient profiling has appeal as a single system for grading foods for the purposes of taxation as well as marketing restrictions. The NBER study supports this approach, finding that taxing nutrients was much better than taxing products if you want to cut calorie intake. A 20% tax on sugar decreased sugar intake by 16.4% and calories by 18.54%. They predicted that nutrient-specific taxes would induce people to buy healthier food.[18]

But what is really needed are real-life examples and these are starting to accumulate. The SHOP study in New Zealand recruited volunteer shoppers who agreed to have their super-market purchases monitored by bar scanners. They were either given tailored education about the food they normally buy, with specific advice on how to choose healthier options for the same (and sometimes a lower) price, or they were given vouchers that effectively dropped the price of the healthy food. The subsidy for the healthy food was 15%, equivalent to GST. To the researchers' surprise and disappointment the sophisticated education program had no effect but there was an 11% increase in fruit and vegetable consumption in response to the 15% drop in price.[19]

The same researchers went on to examine price sensitivity and found (unsurprisingly) that people on lower incomes are more likely to alter what they buy in response to price changes than those on higher incomes and therefore benefit the most from fiscal measures that encourage healthy eating.[20] This is important because taxes on food are usually described by neoliberals as being 'regressive,' meaning that people on low incomes pay relatively more tax than those on higher incomes so any increase in taxation will hit them harder. If, however, the benefits skew in favor of low-income people then you could argue that food tax is 'progressive,' especially if a decrease in inequality follows as a result of less diet-related illness. So whether or not a tax is harmful or helpful depends on what it does to consumption and the size of the price rise has a lot to do with this. Experience with tobacco has taught us that small increases are usually absorbed (smokers just become poorer) but a sharp price rise leads to quitting. Many states in the US apply small taxes to soft drinks and this probably just adds to the grocery bill without affecting sales. In Ireland in the 1980s a 10% rise in price resulted in an 11% fall in soft drink consumption and most public health experts now recommend a 20% tax.[21]

Working to a framework

Governments have a lot of evidence for which public health interventions work and which don't. Then, ideally, policy is developed within an agreed framework—a way of looking at the whole picture. The past master of frameworks is Boyd Swinburn who coined the term 'obesogenic environments' as a description of the collective adverse influences promoting weight gain. He went on to develop the ANGELO (Analysis Grid for Elements Linked to Obesity) framework for analyzing environments for potential barriers to healthy eating and physical activity.[22] But the one I find most useful is a diagram published (by Swinburn and others) in

161

The Lancet series on obesity that categorizes determinants and solutions under the headings of Environments, Behaviours and Physiology.[23]

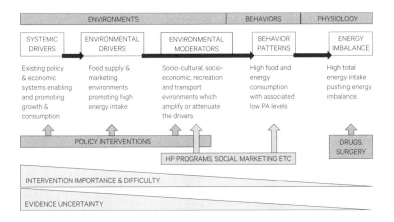

Environmental factors which drive obesity at the macro-economic level appear on the left. To modify these, governments need to address trade agreements and food subsidies which drive overproduction of food. Needless to say, while these interventions are likely to be the most effective there is little real experience to draw on and they are politically difficult. Next along are policy interventions on a national or even local level that alter the availability and marketing of food. This is where the controls on advertising, limits on sites for fast food outlets, and taxes come in. Still politically difficult, and effective. Neoliberal governments are more comfortable operating in the region to the right of this on the diagram. This shows a preoccupation with behavior patterns and attempts to alter these with health promotion and social marketing programs. These initiatives have a low level of political difficulty and efficacy and are resisted by campaigners like me who see them as doing more harm than good. To the very right of the diagram is the non-controversial area in which doctors tinker with physiology using drugs (not very effective) or surgery. Surgery is highly effective for most people who undergo it but as a population intervention it's hopeless as the number of operations required is enormous. The summary of this model is that the easy to implement strategies are those based on personal endeavor but they're ineffective for all but a few.

This model aligns with myriad briefing papers, summit reports, and recommendations from agencies as diverse as the New Zealand Medical Association, the American Heart Association, the World Public Health Nutrition Association, the National Institute for Health and Care Excellence public guidelines group, WHO, the Non Communicable Diseases Alliance, and others, going back over a decade or so. A recent report is from the World Innovation Summit for Health in December 2013.[24] The bottom line in these publications is that the obesity issue needs to be pushed upstream to governments, and is not something that individuals can solve by themselves. It's not even something that the health sector can solve. There is also agreement that dealing with the energy intake side of the equation is the highest priority and this requires policy action on the food supply. A cross-government approach is needed to align policies of agriculture, trade, and health. This isn't to say there's no role for local authorities, schools, workplaces, and parents to support individual endeavour, but the money is on macro-economic policy.

It seems clear that a systems approach is required to deal

with this highly complex problem but time and again I am asked by journalists 'If there was a single thing you could do to treat obesity, what would it be?' My answer is that if we look at the world using a frame of reference of 'improving nutrition' a thousand things would change. Academics are now describing the same approach with a great deal more sophistication. International food policy advisor Corinna Hawkes and others say we need overarching *food policies* with the express aim of improving the human diet. In *The Lancet* series on obesity Hawkes and her group identified four mechanisms through which food policies could influence what we choose to eat.

- By providing an environment that encourages children to learn to prefer healthy food early in life.
- By overcoming barriers such as cost and restricted availability to the expression of healthy food preferences.
- By encouraging people to reassess existing unhealthy preferences when they are choosing and purchasing food using such things as price and presentation (choice architecture).
- By stimulating a food system response as a reaction to policy change. The reformulation of food by manufacturers as a reaction to the ban on trans-fats is an example.

Examples of actions that enhance healthy preference learning

- Protection and promotion of breastfeeding
- Nutrition counseling to pregnant and breastfeeding women
- Teaching of food skills and literacy in schools
- Provision of healthy food in schools
- Reformulation of food intended for children to reduce sugar content
- Subsidization of healthy food for low-income families
- Regulation of unhealthy food to children
- Restricting unhealthy food retail in areas where children gather.[25]

Physical activity at a population level needs to increase and this too requires a cross-governmental approach. Until recently improving health by increasing physical activity has been the preserve of the health sector (and commercial enterprise) with Ministry of Health funding of 'Green Prescriptions' for specific exercise programs and group exercise activities for targeted groups. At the same time the transport sector collects vast amounts of data to analyze the effects of road and pavement sizes, timing of traffic light changes, and so forth to optimize traffic flow. My route to work on foot is dictated partly by where the pedestrian-friendly traffic lights are (good at the bottom of Queen Street, bad at the top of Symonds Street). I've no doubt the same information could optimize the conditions for walking, cycling, and public transport usage, but reducing obesity hasn't been part of the transport sector's mandate. Similarly, the Ministries of

165

Agriculture, and Trade and Enterprise have focused on liberalization of trade to improve export earnings without thought to the health effects of losing food sovereignty.

But where to start? In 2011 the UN sponsored a high-level summit on non-communicable diseases. A timeframe was drawn up for several key goals. By 2013 governments were requested to develop and implement comprehensive strategies to decrease childhood obesity. By 2016 they are to eliminate all forms of marketing, particularly those aimed at children, for foods high in saturated fats, trans-fats, salt, and refined sugars. Regulatory measures to reduce the quantities of fats, sugar, and salt in processed foods were also to be in place by 2013 with the aim of achieving a worldwide salt intake of less than 5 grams per day per capita by 2025.[26] Most countries are well behind schedule.

One way to lead change is to pick the low-hanging fruit and taxing soft drinks may be the place to start. In 2012 the American Public Health Association issued a policy statement recommending a tax on sugar-sweetened beverages.[27] The Rudd Center at Yale regularly monitors public support for this intervention and posted a report of 'The Field Poll' in February 2013: 'Most Californians see a direct linkage between obesity and sugary sodas. Two in three voters support taxing sugar-sweetened beverages if proceeds are tied to improving school nutrition and physical activity programs.'[28] In Ireland a formal health impact report of a proposal to apply a 10% tax to sugar-sweetened beverages indicated this would reduce the number of obese people by 10,000. In response to this the Royal College of Physicians of Ireland wants a 20% tax on sugar-sweetened beverages. France introduced a soda tax in 2012; in January 2014 Mexico introduced a one peso (US7 cents) per litre soda tax; when three month periods of the year before and afterwards were compared the result was a 10% drop in consumption. A year later the liberal city of Berkeley, California, voted for a 1 cent per ounce soda tax and the votes fell just short of supporting the tax in neighboring San Francisco.

Taxing soft drinks may not be the most effective measure to reduce obesity but doing so shifts the focus from personal to societal responsibility. If tobacco control is an accurate example, restoring a healthy default environment will be a long haul and we need to get started now.

Conclusion: *Rise up!*

The obesity epidemic is the result of our obesogenic environment and this can be fixed. But despite all the accumulated evidence there isn't the political will to regulate our environment to favor eating healthily. Some academics are now considering *why* there is such a gap between evidence and policy.[1] For example, do behavioral studies show that decreasing the emphasis on personal responsibility is helpful or harmful in obtaining support for change? The reality is that an environment that is stacked against you living healthily erodes personal freedom and responsibility.[2] Others are analyzing government responses around the world to hold them accountable for (lack of) progress against the WHO obesity and diabetes targets.[3] But perhaps governments are never going to lead the environmental changes needed.

Over the time that I've been writing this book, a subtle shift in public feeling has been taking place in the background and this may overtake and drag anti-obesity measures along with it. Naomi Klein in her terrifying book *This Changes Everything: capitalism vs the climate* describes the failures of unregulated capitalism and how communities, at a grassroots level, are demanding control over their physical environment.[4] This anti-corporate uprising is being led by indigenous peoples around the world in response to such activities as destruction of traditional lands for the purposes of mining or large-scale farming. This echoes the passionate demands for the maintenance of food sovereignty by groups such as La Via Campesina. At the core of peasant movements such as this is an understanding that food is more than just nutrients. Shared meals of traditional food are key to the maintenance of community solidarity and culture. The two movements come together over the issue of diet for a sustainable planet and the term that describes this is 'agroecology.'

Studies have compared the environmental impact of different diets in terms of water and land usage as well as greenhouse gas emissions associated with production and transport. Beef protein is the most expensive food on the planet in terms of methane production and the water and energy costs of feed production. A no-waste, mainly plant-based diet grown locally optimizes health and has minimal impact on the climate. In a largely urban world this goal is being achieved in novel ways. Communal gardens are appearing in parks and on roadside verges and rooftops. In the Canadian city of Laval an acre of rooftop garden produced about 132 tons of greens. In Japan, on a former factory site, a farm the size of a football field produces 10,000 heads of lettuce a day with 80% less food waste and 99% less water than the same volume of food grown in traditional fields.[5] Beehives are increasingly common on city rooftops.

Once you start to grow your own food, wastage becomes abhorrent. Ecologists, epidemiologists, and economists are aligned over the issue of food wastage. By 2050 the population will be 9.3 billion, requiring an extra 6,000 trillion kilocalories a day. Approximately one-third of all food grown ends up in landfill and a quarter of all the water taken and land cleared for the purpose of food production is wasted. Greenhouse gas emissions related to food processing and transport are added to by the effect of rotting food. Just halving the food waste would produce an extra 1314 trillion calories. In the rich global north 42% of food is wasted largely as a result of overconsumption—or buying more than you need. In the poor global south just 17% of available food is wasted, largely at the point of production due to poor transportation and insufficient refrigeration.[6] In the developed world a realization of widespread food wastage has led to programs to redistribute restaurant and supermarket food to those on low incomes, and to voluntary redistribution networks such as the community project in Berlin where refrigerators are available for food donation and communal compost bins deal with anything left over. And then there is 'dumpster-diving,' though this is more political statement than a practical means of sustenance. Freegans (free + vegan) 'forage instead of buying to avoid being wasteful consumers ourselves, to politically challenge the injustice of allowing vital resources to be wasted while multitudes lack basic necessities like food, clothing, and shelter.'[7]

Two articles on news site rabble.ca listed, in March 2015, 10 global food trends. The fifth was the rise of political organizing. The author says that food politics suffers from the classic 'problem of collective action.'[8] It is certainly the case that it's easier to get people to rally around an issue with obvious benefits to their particular group but the realization that civil unrest may be the only way to change the food environment is in itself a significant shift and a cause for optimism. The free market has failed to preserve health and protect the planet and recent protests against free trade agreements in New Zealand show that an intolerance for this is building.

I'd like to see a civil rights uprising that demands an environment where it is easy to eat and exercise in a way that keeps everyone healthy. Those who have most to gain are the people predisposed to obesity and I'd love them to lead this charge. I hope this book gives more strength to their arm.

Epilogue

How to live

I'm a doctor and I spend my days on ward rounds and in diabetes
clinics with people seeking advice for their weight-related medical problems. From the outset I make it clear, for all the reasons
outlined in the book, that I don't expect them to lose weight. I
acknowledge that being overweight is a burden for them and that
of course to be slim would be good for their health. But without an
effective treatment (other than surgery) for obesity, losing weight
can't be part of the therapy. This doesn't mean I don't talk about
diet or exercise, but the emphasis is on optimizing health irrespective of weight.

How to eat

When I talk about diet I don't think it's particularly useful to focus on the things we shouldn't eat. We all know what they are, and if you've inherited the food-seeking genes, you're going to eat them. You *will* eat fries and pizza and donuts and so on. The only exception to this rule is soda. The reason I suggest people don't drink sweetened drinks, apart from the obvious, is because there are artificially sweetened alternatives. I know they're not quite the same, but they're good enough most of the time and it's an easy way to strip a lot of calories out of the diet.

I like to try and persuade people to *add* food to what they usually eat. I tell them about the Finnish Diabetes Prevention Study and the importance of adding extra fiber. This translates to eating natural cereals like porridge oats or unsweetened muesli instead of donuts or pastries for breakfast. I also explain that humans are omnivores designed to forage widely for all of the trace elements we need and that a large number of these come from plants. So we should look for ways to add vegetables and fresh fruit. I'm talking about ordinary fruit and vegetables here—not 'super foods.' This is a marketing term and has nothing to do with our actual nutritional requirements. At the moment people around me are obsessed with 'coconut water.' It drives me nuts. We don't grow coconuts in New Zealand, so this product is packaged, presumably with additives, and flown across the Pacific to be sold in supermarkets. We produce vast amounts of cows' milk in New Zealand and in most places water is delicious straight from the tap. We don't need coconut milk. Kale, almonds, quinoa, and everything else touted as a super food are fads.

If at all practical, I encourage people to cook. Even better is

174

sitting around a table and eating home-cooked food together.
The transformational experience of preparing a meal from raw
ingredients and serving it to others is one of the most deeply satisfying human activities. It doesn't feel quite like that when you
race home from work and have to prepare a meal for your family
night after night, but we need to recognize the value of communal
eating over and above consuming food. Home-cooked meals,
even if they use some processed ingredients, will almost always
be healthier than fast food. We don't add the same salt and sugar
to the food we cook and most of us can't be bothered with deep
frying. Home-prepared lunches win on many levels including
cost. It also means you always have food available, so the moment
your hunger pangs kick in you can reach into your bag for a sandwich, a piece of fruit, or a handful of nuts without resorting to the
candy bar because you don't have time to leave your desk.

If you are incredibly lucky you will have a vegetable garden
or share in a communal garden. Growing your food is another
of those activities that produce pleasure at a deep and primitive
level of our brains. Well, mine anyway. But recommendations to
have a vegetable garden are often made by people who don't actually have one themselves. I have a large garden and it's damned
hard work. Sometimes a storm will blow all the blossoms off your
fruit trees before they're pollinated, caterpillars will destroy
your cabbages, and slugs will eat all of your corn seedlings.
Growing things has given me a deep respect for vegetables and
vegetable-growers and heightened my pleasure in eating season-
ally. Not only are freshly picked vegetables higher in vitamins but
a burgeoning supply of spinach or capsicums or tomatoes will
drive consumption of these things—no gardener can bear to see
food wasted. Even when I lived in an apartment I had tomatoes

growing on the deck in large pots and always had a bay tree and containers of herbs.

Food waste is an issue all on its own because now we are talking about our effect on the planet. Once you get started, it's impossible not to move from food to water and power and packaging. Reducing the amount of processed food we eat ticks all of the boxes nutritionally and environmentally, but really we need to look at meat consumption too. Cutting out one 5 ounce meat meal a week has been calculated to save 430 pounds of carbon dioxide production a year. The numbers are debatable but beef is the most expensive form of protein in terms of environmental impact and, though I'm not vegetarian, I eat little meat and don't buy beef for this reason. Some people have set themselves the challenge of putting nothing into the landfill. This is pretty difficult to achieve, but having this goal drives all sorts of useful behavior change. It means that in addition to not buying bottled water, taking reusable bags to the supermarket, and feeling guilty each time I buy coffee in a paper cup, I make yogurt in a large container that requires one packet instead of buying several small plastic cups. Any leftovers from dinner I freeze or take for lunch and of course I freeze, dehydrate, pickle, and give away excess produce from the garden. I make sourdough bread and leftovers get dried and whizzed for breadcrumbs. Anything organic that doesn't get eaten goes into my compost bin, except for bananas, which I throw in the freezer and when I have three I make a cake. Anyone looking for ideas for using up leftovers and reducing the size of the human footprint on the planet should check out the 1 Million Women Facebook page for inspiration.

On the door of my office is a poster which says:

Food. 1 - Buy it with thought, 2 - Cook it with care, 3 - Use less wheat and meat, 4 - Buy local foods, 5 - Serve just enough, 6 - Use what is left. Don't waste it.

It was produced by the US Food Administration in 1917.

How to be active

There are two distinct aspects of physical activity we need to be aware of. The first is the avoidance of sedentary behavior. If I meet someone who works as a keyboard operator of some sort, a taxi driver, or worst of all, in a call center, I'm worried about the time they spend sitting. I suggest everyone gets up and walks around once an hour. From time to time I chair a session at a conference and typically these will last for 2–3 hours. At some point between speakers I've taken to asking the audience to stand up and move around. They look bemused and a bit embarrassed at first but then they laugh, stand, and stretch and seem more cheerful and alert as a result of the break. My husband is a writer and sits on a Swiss ball to work but these are pretty big and not practical for most workplaces. Some organizations offer standing desks and I rather like the sound of this but you need to have an adjustable computer so that you can sit when you get tired. It's more practical to do as our administration staff at the diabetes center do and have a wall chart of exercises to be done once an hour or to take every opportunity to leave your desk to hand deliver a message or talk to someone in person. Most importantly, you shouldn't lie on the couch watching TV for two or three hours at a stretch after dinner.

If you are going to take up a new exercise for the purpose of improving fitness anything will do, but walking is likely to be the most sustainable in the long term. Best of all is if you can walk to somewhere you need to go every day. This can be to work, to the train station, to the shops. I remind my very overweight patients that you burn up a lot more calories moving a heavy weight and that a slim person will need to walk a lot farther to get the same benefit as they will from a short walk. Perhaps because I care for so many elderly patients who fall I'm increasingly interested in the maintenance of strength and balance as people grow older and encourage exercise for these reasons alone. I promote opportunistic exercise—if there's ever an opportunity to walk somewhere, take it. Especially stairs.

How to treat obesity and diabetes

Treat obesity and diabetes by doing all of the above, plus specific additional treatments. I and others believe that gastric bypass surgery is the best treatment on offer for type 2 diabetes and I wish more people had access to the operation. If you are someone who has inherited the tendency for weight gain and diabetes and you are already very overweight (a BMI of 40 or more), you should be making inquiries about bariatric surgery before you develop the medical problems that make surgery hazardous. Every day on my ward round I see someone in their 50s or 60s with diabetes and cellulitis or sleep apnea or heart failure and I wish they had had bariatric surgery decades earlier.

In terms of medication we know that type 2 diabetes is part of a spectrum of disorders which clump together. I tell people from the outset they will almost certainly need two to three medicines for high blood pressure, another for lipids, quite likely (in New Zealand anyway) gout treatment, and others, in addition to blood sugar lowering agents. So if they have an aversion to taking pills they need to get over it. I also tell them that no matter how careful they are with their diet, even if they do absolutely everything correctly, they will probably need insulin treatment eventually. Too often the threat of insulin is waved like a stick in diabetes clinics and when the pancreas fails the patient feels as though *they* have failed. This is nonsense and ignores the natural history of the disease. I tell them that the good news is that all of these medications are effective and as a result people with diabetes can live long and healthy lives. The single most important thing is to not smoke cigarettes.

How to reduce anti-fat prejudice

Occasionally my views are misinterpreted and I run afoul of the overweight people I want to support. This is because no matter how prevalent it is I don't see excess weight as normal and use the term 'obesity' pathologically. Because of the way it amplifies the risk for such a wide range of illnesses, I think I side with those who call it a disease. We wouldn't dream of blaming or sniggering at someone with eczema or cerebral palsy or epilepsy although perhaps in medieval times they bore the brunt of the prejudice now experienced by the seriously overweight. I make it a mission to describe the biology of obesity in any forum offered and I also disallow any derogatory remarks in my workplace. The young doctors with whom I work are so fastidious in this that they sometimes don't mention weight even in someone admitted with morbid obesity as their main problem. But anti-fat prejudice is deeply entrenched and will take a long time to overturn. I think that making it an issue of human rights may well be required and this will need to be led by those affected (and supported by people like you and me).

How to advocate for a healthy environment

Years before I formed FOE I was on the board of my kids' little primary school. There were many poor families in the area and the kind teachers were in the habit of feeding children cookies when they came to school hungry. These giant cookies were easy to stock in single serves and had a long shelf-life. I expressed my dismay—and to my relief the board members agreed to stock healthier alternatives. They also stopped selling fried fish and chips on the one day of the week children could buy their lunch at school.

I later made a nuisance of myself in the hospital by suggesting we should 'walk the talk' with food for staff and visitors. Sweetened drinks were taken out of all vending machines, ice creams disappeared from the staff cafeteria, and rules put in place for the size of cakes and slices sold in the cafe. At the time this caused a furor and I was threatened with a petition signed by all of the surgeons and anesthetists who wondered 'who the hell I thought I was?' telling people what they could eat. This didn't eventuate and now the Ministry of Health requires all hospitals to have protocols to ensure a healthy food environment for staff. I don't want this to sound easy though, and I still haven't managed to kill off the candy jar that others in my department keep filled for late afternoon sugar fixes.

Another opportunity that comes along from time to time is with the ordering of catering. On any conference committee I like to be involved with the social program. Mostly because I like to organize a good party but also in order to control the menu. I love the Harvard and Massachusetts General Hospital course in internal medicine that's held every June, but on both occasions I attended I was astonished at the terrible food. What are they thinking of serving sweet donuts and pastries for breakfast, soda ad libitum, and on one afternoon, popcorn and chocolate bars? I always provide feedback when invited to and sometimes spontaneously. I have a problem with the way fresh food is packaged and I hate those little stickers on fruit which don't compost. I tend to remove these and apply them to the store container in a small act of protest and I've occasionally removed the plastic wrap and polystyrene tray from the fruit I'm buying and left it at the counter when the wrapping has been especially egregious.

We need to influence the environment over which we have control. For some that will be our own household, but for many it could be our workplace, our local schools, or church. Where I live there's a strong community page on Facebook. It's a great way of mobilizing support, and in addition to matching lost dogs with their owners and exchanging advice on noxious plants we've mounted a successful opposition to the building of a marina and to single-use plastic bags at the supermarket. Once someone put a fake McDonald's sign on a building site near the village and the protests were so violent that McDonald's threatened the prankster with prosecution for bad press. We need to be consistent in our support for changes to the default environment and our resistance to solutions such as free gym memberships or nutrition seminars. This last aspect is terribly important I think. I recently worked with a television crew on a program about obesity and they decided to include a clip on a 'big man's' gym. I had to spell it out to them that this undermined much of what I was saying and reinforced the notion that with the right education/motivation/willpower people could control their weight. *Blocking* the introduction of these initiatives may be as powerful as anything else in getting across the need for environmental controls. Refusing sponsorship from junk food and soda manufacturers gets people thinking too. We are naïve if we think our kids don't develop brand allegiance through iconic imagery on sports equipment and stationery and we need to violently protest whenever a school or workplace accepts funding in this way. I'm embarrassed to say that some years ago we had a McDonald's outlet in the foyer of the children's hospital but the board was shamed into revoking the license.

If nothing else we should try and improve things for the next generation. We should encourage our daughters to eat healthily during pregnancy and to breast feed the baby if at all possible. When grandchildren come to stay we should turn off the television and treat them with a trip to the park, stories read from a book, and home cooking.

Good luck.

Notes

Chapter 1: Does dieting work?

1. MarketsandMarkets. 'Weight Loss and Weight Management Market worth $206.4 Billion by 2019'. MarketsandMarkets, www.marketsandmarkets.com/PressReleases/ weight-loss-obesity-management.asp.
2. Thorkild I. A. Sørensen, et al. 'Intention to lose weight, weight changes, and 18-y mortality in overweight individuals without co-morbidities'. *PLoS Medicine* vol. 2, 2005, e171.
3. Mintel. 'Dieting in 2014? You're not alone – 29 million Brits have tried to lose weight in the last year'. Mintel, 3 January 2014, www.mintel.com/press-centre/ social-and-lifestyle/dieting-in-2014-you-are-not-alone.
4. Robert C. Atkins. *Dr Atkins' Diet Revolution*. New York, David McKay, 1972.
5. Christopher D. Gardner, et al. 'Micronutrient quality of weight-loss diets that focus on macronutrients: results from the A TO Z study'. *American Journal of Clinical Nutrition* vol. 92, 2010, pp. 304–12.
6. Thomas A. Waddeb, Albert J. Stunkard and Kelly D. Brownell. 'Very low calorie diets: their efficacy, safety, and future'. *Annals of Internal Medicine* vol. 99, 1983, pp. 675–84.
7. Michael L. Dansinger, et al. 'Comparison of the Atkins, Ornish, Weight Watchers, and Zone diets for weight loss and heart disease risk reduction: a randomized trial'. *Journal of the American Medical Association* vol. 293, 2005, pp. 43–53.
8. Barbara J. Rolls, Adam Drewnowski and Jenny H. Ledikwe. 'Changing the energy density of the diet as a strategy for weight management'. *Journal of the American Dietetic Association* vol. 105, 2005, pp. 98–103.
9. Charlotte Ayyad and Teis Andersen. 'Long-term efficacy of dietary treatment of obesity: a systematic review of studies published between 1931 and 1999'. *Obesity Reviews* vol. 1, 2000, pp. 113–19.
10. James W. Anderson, et al. 'Long-term weight-loss maintenance: a meta-analysis of US studies'. *American Journal of Clinical Nutrition* vol. 74, 2001, pp. 579–84.
11. Thomas A. Wadden, et al. 'Four year weight losses in the Look AHEAD Study: factors associated with long-term success'. *Obesity* vol. 19, 2011, pp. 1987–98.
12. Deepika Laddu, et al. 'A review of evidence-based strategies to treat obesity in adults'. *Nutrition in Clinical Practice* vol. 26, 2011, pp. 512–25.
13. David R. Jacobs Jr. et al. 'Community-wide prevention strategies: evaluation design of the Minnesota Heart Health Program'. *Journal of Chronic Diseases* vol. 39, 1986, pp. 775–88.
14. Robert W. Jeffery. 'Community programs for obesity prevention: the Minnesota Heart Health Program'. *Obesity Research* vol. 3, 1995, pp. 283s–88s.

15. Boyd Swinburn, et al. 'The Pacific Obesity Prevention in Communities project: project overview and methods'. *Obesity Reviews* suppl. 2, 2011, pp. 3–11.

16. Elaine Rush, et al. 'Project Energize: Whole-region primary school nutrition and physical activity programme: evaluation of body size and fitness 5 years after the randomized controlled trial'. *British Journal of Nutrition* vol. 111, 2014, pp. 363–71.

17. Marie Ng, et al. 'Global, regional, and national prevalence of overweight and obesity in children and adults during 1980–2013: a systematic analysis for the Global Burden of Disease Study 2013'. *The Lancet* vol. 384, 2014, pp. 766–81, doi: 10.1016/S0140-6736(14)60460-8.

18. Melanie D. Klok, S. Jakobsdottir and M. L. Drent. 'The role of leptin and ghrelin in the regulation of food intake and body weight in humans: a review'. *Obesity Reviews* vol. 8, 2007, pp. 21–34.

19. Paul S. MacLean, et al. 'Biology's response to dieting: the impetus for weight regain'. *American Journal of Physiology – Regulatory, Integrative and Comparative Physiology* vol. 301, 2011, R581–R600.

20. Priya Sumithran, et al. 'Long-term persistence of hormonal adaptations to weight loss'. *New England Journal of Medicine* vol. 365, 2011, pp. 1597–604.

21. Eric Doucet, et al. 'Appetite after weight loss by energy restriction and a low-fat diet-exercise follow-up'. *International Journal of Obesity and Related Metabolic Disorders* vol. 24, 2000, pp. 906–14.

22. The Diabetes Prevention Program Research Group. 'Reduction in the incidence of type 2 diabetes with lifestyle intervention or metformin'. *New England Journal of Medicine* vol. 346, 2002, pp. 393–403.

23. Diabetes Prevention Program Research Group. '10-year follow-up of diabetes incidence and weight loss in the Diabetes Prevention Program Outcomes Study'. *The Lancet* vol. 374, 2009, pp. 1677–86, doi:10.1016/S0140-6736(09)61457-4.

24. Guangwei Li, et al. 'The long-term effect of lifestyle interventions to prevent diabetes in the China Da Qing Diabetes Prevention Study: a 20-year follow-up study'. *The Lancet* vol. 371, 2008, pp. 1783–89.

Chapter 2: Is exercise the answer?

1. Mayo Foundation for Medical Education and Research. 'How much am I burning?' Mayo Clinic, www.mayoclinic.org/healthy-lifestyle/weight-loss/in-depth/exercise/art-20050999?pg=2<http://www.mayoclinic.org/healthy-lifestyle/weight-loss/in-depth/exercise/art-20050999?pg=2>.

2. Joseph E. Donnelly, et al. 'Aerobic exercise alone results in clinically significant weight loss for men and women: midwest exercise trial 2'. *Obesity* vol. 21, 2013, E219–E228.

3. Kevin Deighton, et al. 'Appetite, energy intake, and PYY3–36 responses to energy-matched continuous exercise and submaximal high-intensity exercise'. *Applied Physiology, Nutrition, and Metabolism* vol. 38, 2013, pp. 947–52.

4. World Health Organization. 'Global recommendations on physical activity for health'. WHO, 2011, http://www.who.int/dietphysicalactivity/pa/en/index.html.

5. Lisa Farrell, et al. 'The socioeconomic gradient in physical inactivity in England'. The Centre for Market and Public Organisation, University of Bristol, working paper no. 13/311, 2013.

6. Jeannine. S. Schiller, et al. 'Summary health statistics for U.S. adults: National Health Interview Survey, 2010'. National Center for Health Statistics, *Vital Health Stat* vol. 10, 2012, pp. 1–207, www.cdc.gov/nchs/data/series/sr_10/sr10_252.pdf.

7. John J. Reilly, et al. 'Physical activity to prevent obesity in young children: cluster randomised controlled trial'. *British Medical Journal* vol. 333, 2006, p. 1041.

8. Terence J. Wilkin, et al. 'Variation in physical activity lies with the child, not his environment: evidence for an "activitystat" in young children (EarlyBird 16)'. *International Journal of Obesity* vol. 30, 2006, pp. 1050–55.

9. Elaine Rush, et al. 'Project Energize: whole-region primary school nutrition and physical activity programme; evaluation of body-size and fitness 5 years after the randomized controlled trial'. *British Journal of Nutrition* vol. 111, 2014, pp. 363–71.

10. Jeremiah N. Morris, et al. 'Coronary heart-disease and physical activity of work'. *The Lancet* vol. 262, 1953, pp. 1053–57.

11. Anthony A. Laverty, et al. 'Active travel to work and cardiovascular risk factors in the United Kingdom'. *American Journal of Preventive Medicine* vol. 45, 2013, pp. 282–88.

12. Gang Hu, et al. 'Occupational, commuting, and leisure-time physical activity in relation to risk for type 2 diabetes in middle-aged Finnish men and women'. *Diabetologia* vol. 46, 2003, pp. 322–29.

13. Lilah M. Besser and Andrew L. Dannenberg. 'Walking to public transit: steps to help meet physical activity recommendations'. *American Journal of Preventive Medicine* vol. 29, 2005, pp. 273–80.

14. David. W. Dunstan and Neville Owen. 'New exercise prescription: don't just sit there: stand up and move more, more often'. Invited commentary on 'Sitting time and all-cause mortality risk in 222,497 Australian adults'. *Archives of Internal Medicine* vol. 172, 2012, pp. 500–01.

15. Taleb A. Alkhajah, et al. 'Sit–stand workstations: a pilot intervention to reduce office sitting time'. *American Journal of Preventive Medicine* vol. 43, 2012, pp. 298–303.

16. Meredith C. Peddie, et al. 'Breaking prolonged sitting reduces postprandial glycemia in healthy, normal-weight adults: a randomized crossover trial'. *American Journal of Clinical Nutrition* vol. 98, 2013, pp. 358–66.

17. Timothy Gill, et al. 'Whole of government obesity preventions: a rapid review'. Sax Institute, 2013, www.saxinstitute.org.au/wp-content/uploads/Whole-of-government-obesity-prevention-interventions.pdf.

18. Adrian Bauman, et al. 'The International Prevalence Study on Physical Activity: results from 20 countries'. *International Journal of Behavioural Nutrition and Physical Activity* vol. 6, 2009, pp. 21–32.

19. John Pucher, et al. 'Walking and cycling to health: a comparative analysis of city, state, and international data. *American Journal of Public Health* vol. 100, 2010, pp. 1986–92.

185

Chapter 3: Can drugs or surgery make us thin?

1. Paul N. Hopkins and Gerald I. Polukoff. 'Risk of valvular heart disease associated with use of fenfluramine'. *BioMed Central Cardiovascular Disorders* vol. 3, 2003, p. 5.
2. Heidi M. Connolly, et al. 'Valvular heart disease associated with fenfluramine–phentermine'. *New England Journal of Medicine* vol. 337, 1997, pp. 581–88.
3. Thomas A. Wadden, et al. 'Weight maintenance and additional weight loss with liraglutide after low-calorie diet-induced weight loss: the SCALE Maintenance randomized study'. *International Journal of Obesity* vol. 37, 2013, pp. 1443–51, doi:10.1038/ijo.2013.120.
4. Arnold J. Kremen, John H. Linner and Charles Nelson. 'An experimental evaluation of the nutritional importance of proximal and sital small intestine'. *Annals of Surgery* vol. 140, 1954, pp. 439–48.
5. Erden Fikri and Robert Cassella. 'Jejunoileal bypass for massive obesity: results and complications in fifty-two patients'. *Annals of Surgery* vol. 179, 1974, p. 460.
6. Stephen N. Joffe. 'Surgical management of morbid obesity'. *Gut* vol. 22, 1981, pp. 242–54.
7. The United Kingdom National Bariatric Surgery Registry. Bariatric surgeon-level outcomes data report, 2 July 2013, nbsr.e-dendrite.com/.
8. Lars Sjöström. 'Review of the key results from the Swedish Obese Subjects (SOS) trial – a prospective controlled intervention study of bariatric surgery'. *Journal of Internal Medicine* vol. 273, 2013, pp. 219–34.
9. Philip R. Schhauer, et al. 'Bariatric surgery versus intensive medical therapy in obese patients with diabetes'. *New England Journal of Medicine* vol. 366, 2012, pp. 1567–76.
10. Geltrude Mingrone, et al. 'Bariatric surgery versus conventional medical therapy for type 2 diabetes'. *New England Journal of Medicine* vol. 366, 2012, pp. 1577–85.

Chapter 4: Is fatness inherited?

1. Cheryl L. Albright, et al. 'The prevalence of obesity in ethnic admixture adults'. *Obesity* vol. 16, 2008, pp. 1138–43.
2. Albert J. Stunkard, et al. 'An adoption study of human obesity'. *New England Journal of Medicine* vol. 314, 1986, pp. 193–98.
3. Albert J. Stunkard, et al. 'The body-mass index of twins who have been reared apart'. *New England Journal of Medicine* vol. 322, 1990, pp. 1483–87.
4. Hermine H. M. Maes, Michael C. Neale and Lindon J. Eaves. 'Genetic and environmental factors in relative body weight and human adiposity'. *Behavior Genetics* vol. 27, 1997, pp. 325–51.
5. Jane Wardle, et al. 'Evidence for a strong genetic influence on childhood adiposity despite the force of the obesogenic environment'. *American Journal of Clinical Nutrition* vol. 87, 2008, pp. 398–404.

6. Ann M. Ingalls, Margaret M. Dickie and George D. Shell. 'Obese, a new mutation in the house mouse'. *Journal of Heredity* vol. 41, 1950, pp. 317–18.

7. Douglas. L. Coleman. 'Effects of parabiosis of obese with diabetes and normal mice'. *Diabetologia* vol. 9, 1973, pp. 294–98.

8. Yiying Zhang, et al. 'Positional cloning of the mouse obese gene and its human homologue'. *Nature* vol. 372, 1994, pp. 425–32.

9. Jeffrey L. Halaas, et al. 'Weight-reducing effects of the plasma protein encoded by the obese gene'. *Science* vol. 269, 1995, pp. 543–46.

10. William T. Gibson, et al. 'Congenital leptin deficiency due to homozygosity for the Delta133G mutation: report of another case and evaluation of response to four years of leptin therapy'. *Journal of Clinical Endocrinology and Metabolism* vol. 89, 2004, pp. 4821–26.

11. I. Sadaf Farooqi, et al. 'Clinical spectrum of obesity and mutations in the melanocortin 4 receptor gene'. *New England Journal of Medicine* vol. 348, 2003, pp. 1085–95.

12. Timothy M. Frayling, et al. 'A common variant in the FTO gene is associated with body mass index and predisposes to childhood and adult obesity'. *Science* vol. 316, 2007, pp. 889–94.

13. Ali R. Keramati, et al. 'A form of the metabolic syndrome associated with mutations in DYRK1B'. *New England Journal of Medicine* vol. 370, 2014, pp. 1909–19.

14. Adam E. Locke, et al. 'Genetic studies of body mass index yield new insights for obesity biology'. *Nature* vol. 518, 2015, pp. 197–206.

15. Clare. H. Llewellyn, et al. 'Finding the missing heritability in pediatric obesity: the contribution of genome-wide complex trait analysis'. *International Journal of Obesity* vol. 37, 2013, pp. 1506–509.

16. Eleanor Wheeler, et al. 'Genome-wide SNP and CNV analysis identifies common and low-frequency variants associated with severe early-onset obesity'. *Nature Genetics* vol. 45, 2013, pp. 513–17.

17. Tessa J. Roseboom, et al. 'Coronary heart disease after prenatal exposure to the Dutch famine, 1944–45'. *Heart* vol. 84, 2000, pp. 595–98.

18. Gian-Paolo Ravelli, Zena A. Stein and Mervyn W. Susser. 'Obesity in young men after famine exposure in utero and early infancy'. *New England Journal of Medicine* vol. 295, 1976, pp. 349–53.

19. Dana Dabelea, et al. 'Intrauterine exposure to diabetes conveys risks for type 2 diabetes and obesity: a study of discordant sibships'. *Diabetes* vol. 49, 2000, pp. 2208–11.

20. John G. Kral, et al. 'Large maternal weight loss from obesity surgery prevents transmission of obesity to children who were followed for 2 to 18 years'. *Pediatrics* vol. 118, 2006, e1644–e1649.

21. Elmar W. Tobi, et al. 'DNA methylation differences after exposure to prenatal famine are common and timing- and sex-specific'. *Human Molecular Genetics* vol. 18, 2009, pp. 4046–53.

22. James V. Neel. 'Diabetes mellitus: a "thrifty" genotype rendered detrimental by "progress"?' *American Journal of Human Genetics* vol. 14, 1962, p. 353.

23. Jane Wardle, et al. 'Obesity associated genetic variation in FTO is associated with diminished satiety'. *Journal of Clinical Endocrinology and Metabolism* vol. 93, 2008, pp. 3640–43.

24. Larry S. Webber, et al. 'Eating behaviour and weight in children'. *International Journal of Obesity* vol. 33, 2008, pp. 21–28.

25. Clare H. Llewellyn, et al. 'Inherited behavioral susceptibility to adiposity in infancy: a multivariate genetic analysis of appetite and weight in the Gemini birth cohort'. *American Journal of Clinical Nutrition* vol. 95, 2012, pp. 633–39.

26. Lester B. Salans, Edward S. Horton and Ethan A. H. Sims. 'Experimental obesity in man: cellular character of the adipose tissue'. *Journal of Clinical Investigation* vol. 50, 1971, pp. 1005–11.

27. James A. Levine, Norman L. Eberhardt and Michael D. Jensen. 'Role of nonexercise activity thermogenesis in resistance to fat gain in humans'. *Science* vol. 283, 1999, pp. 212–14.

28. Fabrizio Pasanisi, et al. 'Evidence of brown fat activity in constitutional leanness'. *Journal of Clinical Endocrinology and Metabolism* vol. 98, 2013, pp. 1214–18.

29. Georgirene D. Vladutiu and Elizabeth Tabone. Correspondence. 'Mitochondrial Disease in Patients with Exercise Intolerance'. *New England Journal of Medicine* vol. 342, 2000, pp. 438–40.

30. Matthieu Million and Didier Raoult. 'The role of the manipulation of the gut microbiota in obesity'. *Current Infectious Disease Reports* vol. 15, 2013, pp. 25–30.

31. Kyle J. Wolf and Robin G. Lorenz. 'Gut microbiota and obesity'. *Current Obesity Reports* vol. 1, 2012, pp. 1–8.

32. Eileen F. Murphy, et al. 'Divergent metabolic outcomes arising from targeted manipulation of the gut microbiota in diet-induced obesity'. *Gut* vol. 62, 2013, pp. 220–26.

33. Julia K. Goodrich, et al. 'Human genetics shape the gut microbiome'. *Cell* vol. 159, 2014, pp. 789–99.

34. Marko Kalliomäki, et al. 'Early differences in fecal microbiota composition in children may predict overweight'. *American Journal of Clinical Nutrition* vol. 87, 2008, pp. 534–38.

35. Eric Ravussin and Clifton Bogardus. 'Energy balance and weight regulation: genetics versus environment'. *British Journal of Nutrition* vol. 83, 2000, S17–S20.

Chapter 5: How new ways of living have led to new ways of eating

1. Darius Lakdawalla and Tomas Philipson. 'The growth of obesity and technological change'. *Economics and Human Biology* vol. 7, 2009, pp. 283–93.

2. Statistics New Zealand. 'Household spending compared with 40 years ago'. Statistics New Zealand, 28 November 2013, http://m.stats.govt.nz/browse_for_stats/ people_and_communities/Households/40years-hes-infographic.

3. Joseph Schmidhuber and Prakash Shetty. 'Nutrition transition, obesity and noncommunicable diseases: drivers, outlook and concerns'. *SCN News* vol. 29, 2005, pp. 13–19.

4. Transport Monitoring Team, Ministry of Transport. 'How New Zealanders travel: trends in New Zealand household travel 1989–2008'. Ministry of Transport, Wellington, 2009, p. 4.

5. Fahui Wang, Ming Wen and Yanqing Xu. 'Population-adjusted street connectivity, urbanicity and risk of obesity in the US'. *Applied Geography* vol. 41, 2013, pp. 1–14.

6. Paul Mees and Jago Dodson. 'Backtracking Auckland: bureaucratic rationality and public preferences in transport planning'. Urban Research Program, Griffiths University, issue paper 5, 2006.

7. Ministry of Transport. *The New Zealand Transport Strategy 2008*. Ministry of Transport, 2008, www.transport.govt.nz/ourwork/Pages/AppendixC-TheNewZealandTransportStrategy.aspx.

8. Ministry for the Environment. 'Vehicle kilometres travelled by road'. Ministry for the Environment, environmental report card, March 2009, www.mfe.govt.nz/environmental-reporting/transport/vehicle-km-travelled/total-vkt/.

9. Joyce Dargay and Dermot Gately. 'Income's effect on car and vehicle ownership, worldwide: 1960–2015'. *Transportation Research Part A: Policy and Practice* vol. 33, 1999, pp. 101–38.

10. 'The future of driving: Seeing the back of the car'. *Economist* 22 September 2012, www.economist.com/node/21563280.

11. Meizi He, et al. 'The influence of local food environments on adolescents' food purchasing behaviors'. *International Journal of Environmental Research and Public Health* vol. 9, 2012, pp. 1458–71.

12. Ann Forsyth, et al. 'Do adolescents who live or go to school near fast-food restaurants eat more frequently from fast-food restaurants?' *Health and Place* vol. 18.6, 2012, pp. 1261–69.

13. Common Sense Media. 'How much screen time is OK for my kid(s)?' Common Sense Media, www.commonsensemedia.org/screen-time/how-much-screen-time-is-ok-for-my-kids.

14. MedlinePlus Medical Encyclopedia. 'Screen time and children'. National Institute of Health, www.nlm.nih.gov/medlineplus/ency/patientinstructions/000355.htm.

15. Carlos J. Crespo, et al. 'Television watching, energy intake, and obesity in US children: results from the third National Health and Nutrition Examination Survey, 1988–1994'. *Archives of Pediatrics and Adolescent Medicine* vol. 155, 2001, pp. 360–65.

16. Jennifer Utter, Robert Scragg and David Schaaf. 'Associations between television viewing and consumption of commonly advertised foods among New Zealand children and young adolescents'. *Public Health Nutrition* vol. 9, 2006, pp. 606–12.

17. Kristen L. Knutson, et al. 'The metabolic consequences of sleep deprivation'. *Sleep Medicine Reviews* vol. 11, 2007, pp. 163–78.

18. Eric Schlosser. *Fast Food Nation: The dark side of the all-American meal*. New York, Houghton Mifflin Harcourt, 2001.

189

19. Colleen M. Doak, et al. 'The dual burden household and the nutrition transition paradox'. *International Journal of Obesity* vol. 29, 2005, pp. 129–36.

20. Barry M. Popkin and Samara Joy Nielsen. 'The sweetening of the world's diet'. *Obesity Research* vol. 11, 2003, pp. 1325–32.

21. Josef Schmidhuber and Prakash Shetty. 'The nutrition transition to 2030. Why developing countries are likely to bear the major burden'. *Acta Agriculturae Scand* Section c 2.3–4, 2005, pp. 150–66.

22. Carlos Augusto Monteiro, et al. 'Increasing consumption of ultra-processed foods and likely impact on human health: evidence from Brazil'. *Public Health Nutrition* vol. 14, 2011, p. 7.

23. Statistics New Zealand. 'Retail Trade Survey: December 2014 quarter'. Statistics New Zealand, 16 February 2015, www.stats.govt.nz/browse_for_stats/industry_sectors/RetailTrade/RetailTradeSurvey_HOTPDec14qtr/Commentary.aspx.

24. Nelson Lichtenstein (ed.). *Wal-Mart: The face of twenty-first-century capitalism*. New York, The New Press, 2013.

25. Tescopoly. 'Issues and impacts'. Tescopoly, www.tescopoly.org/issues-and-impacts.

26. Marion Nestle. 'Why are so many Americans overweight?' IIP Digital, 22 November 2010, iipdigital.usembassy.gov/st/english/publication/2010/11/20101122114827noiram0.1394573.html#axzz3t1rpgmXp.

Chapter 6: How the economics of food puts more of it on our plates

1. Philip James. 'World agriculture, food and nutrition policy. Government for the people [As I see it]'. *World Nutrition* vol. 4, 2013, pp. 342–58.

2. J. M. Harries and Dorothy F. Hollingsworth. 'Food supply, body weight, and activity in Great Britain, 1943–9'. *British Medical Journal* vol. 1, 1953, p. 75.

3. Mary Francis Kennedy Fisher. *How to Cook a Wolf*. New York, North Point Press, 1942.

4. Marion Nestle. *Food Politics: How the food industry influences nutrition and health*. 3rd edition. Berkley and Los Angeles, University of California Press, 2013.

5. Mike Russo and Dan Smith. 'Apples to Twinkies 2013: comparing taxpayer subsidies for fresh produce and junk food'. U.S. PIRG, 2013, www.uspirg.org/reports/usp/apples-twinkies-2013.

6. Ibid.

7. Judy Putnam, Jane Allshouse and Linda Scott Kantor. 'US per capita food supply trends: more calories, refined carbohydrates, and fats'. *Food Review* vol. 25, 2002, pp. 2–15.

8. David Wallinga. 'Today's food system: how healthy is it?' *Journal of Hunger and Environmental Nutrition* vol. 4, 2009, pp. 251–81.

9. Liselotte Schäfer Elinder. 'Obesity, hunger, and agriculture: the damaging role of subsidies'. *British Medical Journal* vol. 331, 2005, pp. 1333–36.

10. Nikos Alexandratos and Jelle Bruinsma. 'World agriculture towards 2030/2050: the 2012 revision'. ESA working paper no. 12-03. Rome, Food and Agriculture Organization of the United Nations, 2013.
11. National Corn Growers Association. 'World of corn 2013'. National Corn Growers Association, 2013, www.ncga.com/upload/files/documents/pdf/WOC%202012.pdf.
12. Michael Pollan. *The Omnivore's Dilemma: A natural history of four meals*. New York, Penguin, 2006.
13. David Pimentel, Tad Patzek and Gerald Cecil. 'Ethanol production: energy, economic, and environmental losses'. *Reviews of Environmental Contamination and Toxicology*. New York, Springer, 2007, pp. 25–41.
14. Geof Rayner, et al. 'Trade liberalization and the diet transition: a public health response'. *Health Promotion International* vol. 21, 2006, pp. 67–74.
15. Andrea Brower. 'Food, farmers and the TPP'. Scoop, 3 June 2012, www.scoop.co.nz/stories/HL1206/S00005/food-farmers-and-the-tpp.htm.
16. 'Samoa seeks ban on fatty meat imports'. *Samoa Observer*, 17 May 2013, www.samoaobserver.ws/other/food/4875-samoa-seeks-ban-on-fatty-meat-imports.
17. 'Samoa lifts ban on high-fat turkey tails'. ABC News, 20 May 2013, www.abc.net.au/news/2013-05-20/an-samoa-lifts-ban-on-high-fat-turkey-tails/4699506.
18. Mike Evans, et al. 'Globalization, diet, and health: an example from Tonga'. *Bulletin of the World Health Organization* vol. 79, 2001, pp. 856–62.
19. Oliver Nieburg. 'Mondelez creates $600m kitty to seize emerging markets'. Confectionery News.com, 30 May 2013, www.confectionerynews.com/Manufacturers/Mondelez-creates-600m-kitty-to-seize-emerging-markets.
20. Karen Lock, et al. 'Potential causes and health effects of rising global food prices'. *British Medical Journal* vol. 339, 2009, p. 2403.
21. Paul Nicholson. 'La Via Campesina. The revolt of the peasants'. Commentary. *World Nutrition* vol. 4, 2013, www.wphna.org/htdocs/2013_feb_wn3_campesina.htm.

Chapter 7: How we're sold on junk food

1. Eric Schlosser. *Fast Food Nation: The dark side of the all-American meal*. New York, Houghton Mifflin Harcourt, 2001.
2. Gareth Morgan and Geoff Simmons. *Appetite for Destruction: Food – the good, bad and the fatal*. Wellington, The Public Interest Publishing Company, 2013.
3. Nadia Slimani, et al. 'Contribution of highly industrially processed foods to the nutrient intakes and patterns of middle-aged populations in the European Prospective Investigation into Cancer and Nutrition study'. *European Journal of Clinical Nutrition* vol. 63, 2009, S206–S225.
4. Janet Hoek. 'Marketing communications and obesity: a view from the dark side'. *Journal of the New Zealand Medical Association* vol. 118, 2005, pp. 8–11.
5. 'Tesco petrol stations use face-scan tech to target ads'. BBC, 4 November 2013, www.bbc.com/news/technology-24803378.

6. Mary-Ann Carter, et al. 'Food, fizzy, and football: promoting unhealthy food and beverages through sport – a New Zealand case study'. *BioMed Central Public Health* vol. 13, 2013, p. 126.

7. Marie A. Bragg, et al. 'Athlete endorsements in food marketing'. *Pediatrics* vol. 132, 2013, pp. 805–10.

8. Lisa M. Powell, et al. 'Trends in the nutritional content of TV food advertisements seen by children in the US: analyses by age, food categories and companies'. *Archives of Pediatrics and Adolescent Medicine* vol. 165, 2011, pp. 1078–86.

9. Frans Folkvord, et al. 'Impulsivity, "advergames", and food intake'. *Pediatrics* vol. 133, 2014, pp. 1007–12.

10. Jennifer L. Harris, et al. *Fast Food FACTS 2013: Measuring progress in nutrition and marketing to children and teens.* Yale Rudd Center for Food Policy and Obesity, 2013, www.fastfoodmarketing.org/media/FastFoodFACTS_report.pdf.

11. Banksy. *Cut It Out.* Weapons of Mass Disruption, 2004.

12. Cliona Ni Mhurchu and Delvina Gorton. 'Nutrition labels and claims in New Zealand and Australia: a review of use and understanding'. *Australian and New Zealand Journal of Public Health* vol. 31, 2007, pp. 105–12.

13. John White, George Thomson and Louise Signal. 'Front-of-pack nutrition labelling: where to now'. *Journal of the New Zealand Medical Association* vol. 123, 2010, pp. 12–16.

14. Sandra Jones. 'Fat free and 100% natural: seven food labelling tricks exposed'. *The Conversation*, 11 April 2014, Theconversation.com/fat-free-and-100-natural-seven-food-labelling-tricks-exposed-25143.

15. Mike Rayner, Peter Scarborough and Asha Kaur. 'Nutrient profiling and the regulation of marketing to children. Possibilities and pitfalls'. *Appetite* vol. 62, 2013, pp. 232–35.

16. Brussels Sunshine. 'High time for CIAA to come clean on its lobbying'. *Brussels Sunshine*, 23 June 2010, blog.brusselssunshine.eu/2010/06/high-time-for-ciaa-to-come-clean-on-its.html.

17. Corporate Europe Observatory. 'Food lobby bashes MEPs on labelling'. Corporate Europe Observatory, 17 April 2011, Corporateeurope.org/2011/04/food-lobby-bashes-meps-labelling.

18. Marion Nestle. *Food Politics: How the food industry influences nutrition and health.* 3rd edition. Berkeley and Los Angeles, University of California Press, 2013.

19. Michele Simon. 'Best public relations that money can buy: a guide to food industry front groups'. Center for Food Safety, 2013, www.centerforfoodsafety.org/files/front_groups_final_84531.pdf.

20. Edward Archer, Gregory A. Hand and Steven N. Blair. 'Validity of US nutritional surveillance: National Health and Nutrition Examination Survey caloric energy intake data, 1971–2010'. *PloS One* vol. 8, 2013, e76632.

21. Marion Nestle. 'Annal of Nutrition Science: Coca-Cola 1; NHANES 0'. *Food Politics*, 14 October 2013, www.foodpolitics.com/2013/10/annals-of-nutrition-science-coca-cola-1nhanes-0/.

22. Lisa Te Morenga, Simonette Mallard and Jim Mann. 'Dietary sugars and body weight:

systematic review and meta-analyses of randomised controlled trials and cohort studies'. *British Medical Journal* vol. 346, 2013, pp. 1–25.

23. Kathryn A. Kaiser, et al. 'Will reducing sugar-sweetened beverage consumption reduce obesity? Evidence supporting conjecture is strong, but evidence when testing effect is weak'. *Obesity Reviews* vol. 14, 2013, pp. 620–33, doi:10.1111/obr.12048.

24. Maira Bes-Rastrollo, et al. 'Financial conflicts of interest and reporting bias regarding the association between sugar-sweetened beverages and weight gain: A systematic review of systematic reviews'. *PLoS Medicine* vol. 10, 2013, e1001578.

25. Nicky Hager. *Dirty Politics: How attack politics is poisoning New Zealand's political environment*. Nelson, Craig Potton Publishing, 2014.

26. Kate Geary. '"Our Land, Our Lives": Time out on the global land rush'. Oxfam Briefing Note, October 2012, www.oxfam.org/sites/www.oxfam.org/files/bn-land-lives-freeze-041012-en_1.pdf.

27. Greenpeace. 'Palm kernel expellar Q & A for media'. Greenpeace, www.greenpeace.org.nz/fonterra/GREENPEACEPalmkernelQ&A.pdf.

28. Vasanti S. Malik and Frank B. Hu. 'Sweeteners and risk of obesity and type 2 diabetes: the role of sugar-sweetened beverages'. *Current Diabetes Reports* vol. 12, 2012, pp. 195–203.

29. Michele Simon. 'Super-sized lies: why you can't trust promises by McDonald's'. *Huffington Post*, 9 October 2013, www.huffingtonpost.com/michele-simon/supersized-lies_b_4064984.html.

30. Kelly D. Brownell. 'Thinking forward: the quicksand of appeasing the food industry'. *PLoS Medicine* vol. 9, 2012, e1001254.

31. Aseem Malhotra. 'Food giants, not magazine diets, endanger your health'. *The Guardian*, 30 December 2012, www.theguardian.com/commentisfree/2012/dec/30/add-weight-fight-food-giants.

32. Derek Yach. 'Can we leave industry to lead efforts to improve population health? Yes'. *British Medical Journal* vol. 346, 2013, f2279.

33. David Stuckler and Marion Nestle. 'Big food, food systems, and global health'. *PLoS Medicine* vol. 9, 2012, e1001242.

34. Jane Martin. 'Hungry Jack's flouts advertising standards', *Crikey*, 4 February 2010, www.crikey.com.au/2010/02/04/hungry-jacks-flouts-advertising-standards/.

35. Oliver Nieburg. 'Hershey marks biggest outlay in Asia with $250m Malaysia plant'. Food Navigator-Asia, 4 October 2013, www.foodnavigator-asia.com/content/view/print/829136.

Chapter 8: How the overweight are stigmatized

1. Cynthia L. Ogden, et al. 'Obesity and socioeconomic status in children and adolescents: United States, 2005–2008'. National Center for Health Statistics, *NCHS Data Brief* no. 51, 2010, www.cdc.gov/nchs/data/databriefs/db51.pdf.

2. National Poverty Center. 'Poverty in the United States: frequently asked questions'.

National Poverty Center, The University of Michigan Gerald R. Ford School of Public Policy, www.npc.umich.edu/poverty/#2.

3. Child Poverty Monitor. 'Child poverty and living standards'. The Children's Social Health Monitor, New Zealand, www.nzchildren.co.nz/PovertyIntroduction.php.

4. Tasileta Teevale, et al. 'The role of sociocultural factors in obesity and aetiology in Pacific adolescents and their parents: a mixed-methods study in Auckland, New Zealand'. *New Zealand Medical Journal* vol. 123, 2010, pp. 26–36.

5. Jamie Pearce, et al. 'Neighbourhood deprivation and access to fast-food retailing: a national study'. *American Journal of Preventive Medicine* vol. 32, 2007, pp. 375–82.

6. Dianna M. Smith, et al. 'Neighbourhood food environment and area deprivation: spatial accessibility to grocery stores selling fresh fruit and vegetables in urban and rural settings'. *International Journal of Epidemiology* vol. 39, 2010, pp. 277–84.

7. Andrea S. Richardson, et al. 'Are neighbourhood food resources distributed inequitably by income and race in the USA? Epidemiological findings across the urban spectrum'. *British Medical Journal Open*, vol. 2, 2012, e000698, doi: 10.1136/bmjopen-2011-000698.

8. Tatiana Anreyeva, Michael W. Long and Kelly D. Brownell. 'The impact of food prices on consumption: a systematic review of research on the price elasticity of demand for food'. *American Journal of Public Health* vol. 100, 2010, pp. 216–22.

9. Sarah Boseley. 'Mexican soda tax cuts sales of sugary soft drinks by 6% in first year'. *The Guardian*, 18 June 2015, www.theguardian.com/world/2015/jun/18/mexican-soda-tax-cuts-sales-first-year.

10. Adam Drenowski. 'Obesity and the food environment: dietary energy and diet costs'. *American Journal of Preventive Medicine* vol. 27, supplement 10, 2004, pp. 154–62.

11. Trenton G. Smith, Christiana Stoddart and Michael G. Barnes. 'Why the poor get fat: weight gain and economic insecurity'. *Forum for Health Economics and Policy* vol. 12, 2009, pp. 1–31.

12. Steven H. Woolf, et al. 'Citizen centred health promotion: building collaborations to facilitate healthy living'. *American Journal of Preventive Medicine* vol. 40, supplement 1, 2011, S38–S47.

13. Ahmedin Jemal, et al. 'Mortality from leading causes and race in the United States, 2001'. *American Journal of Preventive Medicine* vol. 34, 2008, pp. 1–8.

14. Shobhana Ramachandran, et al. 'Expenditure on health care incurred by diabetes subjects in a developing country – a study from southern India'. *Diabetes Research and Clinical Practice* vol. 48, 2000, pp. 37–42.

15. Alistair Woodward and Tony Blakely. *The Healthy Country? A history of life and death in New Zealand*. Auckland, Auckland University Press, 2014.

16. Y. Claire Wang, et al. 'Health and economic burden of the projected obesity trends in the USA and the UK'. *The Lancet* vol. 378, 2011, pp. 815–25.

17. Anita L. M. Moodie, et al. 'Health care and lost productivity costs of overweight and obesity in New Zealand'. *Australian and New Zealand Journal of Public Health* vol. 36, 2012, pp. 550–56.

18. Rebecca M. Puhl and Chelsea A. Heuer. 'The stigma of obesity: a review and update'. *Obesity* vol. 5, 2009, pp. 941–64.

19. John Cawley. 'The impact of obesity on wages'. *Journal of Human Resources* vol. 39, 2004, pp. 451–74.

20. Cheryl L. Maranto and Ann F. Stenoien. 'Weight discrimination: a multidisciplinary analysis'. *Employee Responsibility and Rights Journal* vol. 12, 2000, pp. 9–24.

21. Rebecca M. Puhl and Kelly D. Brownell. 'Confronting and coping with weight stigma: an investigation of overweight and obese individuals'. *Obesity* vol. 14, 2006, pp. 1802–15.

22. Janet D. Latner and Albert Stunkard. 'Getting worse: the stigmatization of obese children'. *Obesity Research* vol. 11, 2003, pp. 452–56.

23. Andrew J. Hill and E. K. Silver. 'Fat, friendless and unhealthy: 9-year old children's perception of body shape stereotypes'. *International Journal of Obesity and Related Metabolic Disorders* vol. 19, 1995, pp. 423–40.

24. Richard M. Lerner and Elizabeth Gellert. 'Body build identification, preference, and aversion in children'. *Developmental Psychology* vol. 1, 1995, pp. 456–62.

25. Christian S. Crandall. 'Do parents discriminate against their heavyweight daughters?' *Personality and Social Psychology Bulletin* vol. 21, 1991, pp. 724–35.

26. Lenny R. Vartanian. 'Disgust and perceived control in attitudes towards obese people'. *International Journal of Obesity* vol. 34, 2010, pp. 1302–07.

27. Kerry S. O'Brien, et al. 'Reducing anti-fat prejudice in pre-service health students: a randomized trial'. *Obesity* vol. 18, 2010, pp. 2138–44, doi: 10.1038/oby.2010.79.

28. Lindsay F. Wiley. 'Shame, blame, and the emerging law of obesity control'. *University of California Davis Law Review* vol. 47, 2013, pp. 121–88.

29. Rebecca. M. Puhl and Chelsea A. Heuer. 'Obesity stigma: Important considerations for public health'. *Framing Health Matters. American Journal of Public Health* vol. 100, 2010, pp. 1019–28.

Chapter 9: How governments can flick the switch

1. Nicole L. Novak and Kelly D. Brownell. 'Role of policy and government in the obesity epidemic'. *Circulation* vol. 126, 2012, pp. 2345–52.

2. Richard H. Thaler and Cass R. Sunstein. *Nudge: Improving decisions about health, wealth, and happiness.* New Haven & London, Yale University Press, 2008, p. 6.

3. Robert Baldwin. 'From regulation to behaviour change: giving nudge the third degree'. *Modern Law Review* vol. 77, 2014, pp. 831–57.

4. Theresa M. Marteau, et al. 'Judging nudging: can nudging improve population health?' *British Medical Journal* vol. 342, 2011, pp. 263–65.

5. Adam Oliver, Geof Rayner and Tim Lang. 'Is nudge an effective public health strategy to tackle obesity? No'. *British Medical Journal* vol. 342, 2011 d2177, doi: 10.1136/bmj.d2177.

6. Barry McCormick and I. Stone. 'Economic costs of obesity and the case for government intervention'. *Obesity Reviews* vol. 8, 2007, pp. 161–64.

7. Anthony Rodgers, et al. 'Distribution of major health risks: findings from the Global Burden of Disease study'. *PLoS Medicine* vol. 1, 2004, e27.

8. John Cawley and Chad Meyerhoefer. 'The medical care costs of obesity: an instrumental variables approach'. *Journal of Health Economics* vol. 31, 2012, pp. 219–30.

9. David E. Bloom, et al. 'The global economic burden of noncommunicable diseases'. Program on the Global Demography of Aging, working paper no. 8712, 2012.

10. Colin Bos, et al. 'Understanding consumer acceptance of intervention strategies for healthy food choices: a qualitative study'. *BioMed Central Public Health* vol. 3, 2013, p. 1073.

11. Robert W. Jeffery. 'Community programs for obesity prevention: the Minnesota Heart Health Program'. *Obesity Research* vol. 3, 1995, pp. 283s–88s.

12. Janet Currie, et al. 'The effect of fast food restaurants on obesity and weight gain'. National Bureau of Economic Research, working paper no. w14721, 2009.

13. Prabhat Jha and Frank J. Chaloupka. *Tobacco Control in Developing Countries*. Oxford University Press, 2000.

14. Randy W. Elder, et al. 'The effectiveness of tax policy interventions for reducing excessive alcohol consumption and related harms.' *American Journal of Preventive Medicine* vol. 38, 2010, pp. 217–29.

15. Michele Cecchini, et al. 'Tackling of unhealthy diets, physical inactivity, and obesity: health effects and cost-effectiveness'. *The Lancet* vol. 376, 2010, pp. 1775–84.

16. Michelle M. Haby, et al. 'A new approach to assessing the health benefit from obesity interventions in children and adolescents: the assessing cost-effectiveness in obesity project'. *International Journal of Obesity* vol. 30, 2006, pp. 1463–75.

17. Peter Scarborough, Mike Rayner and Lynn Stockley. 'Developing nutrient profile models: a systematic approach'. *Public Health Nutrition* vol. 10, 2007, pp. 330–36.

18. Matthew Harding and Michael Lovenheim. 'The effect of prices on nutrition: comparing the impact of product-and nutrient-specific taxes'. National Bureau of Economic Research, working paper no. w19781, 2014.

19. Cliona Ni Mhurchu, et al. 'Effects of price discounts and tailored nutrition education on supermarket purchases: a randomized controlled trial'. *American Journal of Clinical Nutrition* vol. 91, 2010, pp. 736–47.

20. Cliona Ni Mhurchu, et al. 'Food prices and consumer demand: differences across income levels and ethnic groups'. *PloS One* vol. 8, 2013, e75934.

21. Oliver T. Mytton, Dushy Clarke and Mike Rayner. 'Taxing unhealthy food and drinks to improve health'. *British Medical Journal* vol. 344, 2012, e2931.

22. Boyd Swinburn, Garry Egger and Fezeela Raza. 'Dissecting obesogenic environments: the development and application of a framework for identifying and prioritizing environmental interventions for obesity'. *Preventive Medicine* vol. 29, 1999, pp. 563–70.

23. Boyd A. Swinburn, et al. 'The global obesity pandemic: shaped by global drivers and local environments'. *The Lancet* vol. 378, 2011, pp. 804–14.

24. The NCD Alliance. 'Proposed outcomes document for the United Nations High-Level Summit on Non-Communicable Diseases'. The NCD Alliance, 2011.

25. Corinna Hawkes, et al. 'Smart food policies for obesity prevention'. *The Lancet* vol. 385, 2015, pp. 2410–21.

26. Shiriki Kumanyika, Kimberley Libman and Ana Garcia. 'Strategic action to combat the obesity epidemic'. Report of the Obesity Working Group, World Innovation Summit for Health, Doha, Qatar, 10–11 December 2013.

27. American Public Health Association. 'Taxes on sugar-sweetened beverages'. American Public Health Association, policy statement 2012, 30 October 2012.

28. Mark DiCamillo and Mervin Field. 'Most Californians see a direct linkage between obesity and sugary sodas. Two in three voters support taxing sugar-sweetened beverages if proceeds are tied to improving school nutrition and physical activity programs'. The Field Poll, release # 2436, Field Research Corporation, 14 February 2013, www.field.com/fieldpollonline/subscribers/Rls2436.pdf.

Conclusion: Rise up!

1. Kelly D. Brownell and Christina A. Roberto. 'Strategic science with policy impact'. *The Lancet* vol. 385, 2015, pp. 2445–46, doi: 10.1016/S0140-6736(14)62397-7.

2. Kelly D. Brownell, et al. 'Personal responsibility and obesity: a constructive approach to a controversial issue'. *Health Affairs* vol. 29, 2010, pp. 379–87.

3. Boyd Swinburn, et al. 'Strengthening of accountability systems to create healthy food environments and reduce global obesity'. *The Lancet* vol. 385, 2015, pp. 2534–45, doi: 10.1016/S0140-6736(14)61747-5.

4. Naomi Klein. *This Changes Everything: capitalism vs the climate*. New York, Simon & Schuster, 2014.

5. Wayne Roberts. 'Five more global food trends for 2015'. Rabble.ca, 13 January 2015, rabble.ca/print/news/2015/01/five-more-global-food-trends-2015.

6. Ibid.

7. 'What is a Freegan?' Freegan.info, freegan.info/.

8. Roberts. 'Five more global food trends.'

Acknowledgments

I'd like to start with the friends and colleagues who encouraged me in my role as an anti-obesity advocate. Sarah Thomson is the most important of these. As CEO of Diabetes New Zealand and a former member of ASH she understood advocacy back when I didn't have a clue what it meant. She was the brains behind FOE (Fight the Obesity Epidemic) and I was the mouth. Those early days were heroic times and we had some terrific adventures and quite a lot of political traction. Robin and John White were early members of the FOE executive and soon became the engine room of the organization. We will all miss Robin's generosity as host (lavish snacks and bottles of wine) at our executive meetings as well as her expertise with managing the website and media enquiries and producing *Obesity News*. Many good people have been members of the executive over the years but most notable is Kris Erickson who joined at the very beginning and has been a source of constant enthusiasm.

Boyd Swinburn is actually responsible for FOE's existence. When I wanted to throw my support behind whoever was doing the best job of campaigning against obesity, Boyd said that Sarah and I needed to form our own organization. So we did. Over the years, Boyd has been a great supporter and it's wonderful to have him back in New Zealand leading obesity research. He is now part of a very large academic community—producing all the evidence a government could possibly need to make meaningful changes to reduce obesity prevalence. I have been very grateful to these public health specialists and researchers for treating me as one of the gang despite my amateur status.

In terms of writing the book, I must thank Sam Elworthy for approaching me many years ago to suggest the project. I completely rejected the notion at first but came around to the idea after years of having long and nuanced interviews with journalists turned into sound bites for 12-year-olds. Sam may have regretted his proposal as he struggled to get me to understand 'passive voice' and turn my rambling prose into something people could read. Thanks for the creative writing course, Sam! I'm amazed at the number of people required to produce a book and my thanks is extended to all of the others who reviewed the manuscript and provided editorial advice, particularly Rebecca Lal.

Most important to me has been the enthusiasm of my family. My daughters Alice and Olivia are fabulous women and both are complete foodies. Alice is a witty writer and craft beer aficionado and Olivia a talented cook and photographer of (mostly wicked) food for her blog 'The Hungry Cook.' John is the real wordsmith of the family—my chatter bears no relationship to his beautifully crafted prose. He was chief gardener and provider of fresh snapper over the time I wrote this. I have my parents Gillian and Ray to thank for their love and loyalty and most importantly for their terrific genes. They are both hale and hearty at 83 and 92, respectively.

Finally, I want to thank my patients. All doctors learn most from the people they treat but obese people are often shy and many have learned not to trust doctors. I hope they feel I have represented them honestly and that this book is a tribute to them.

Index